Principles and Practice of
Percutaneous Tracheostomy

Principles and Practice of Percutaneous Tracheostomy

SP Ambesh

Professor and Senior Consultant
Department of Anaesthesiology
Sanjay Gandhi Postgraduate Institute of Medical Sciences
Lucknow (India)

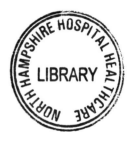

JAYPEE BROTHERS MEDICAL PUBLISHERS (P) LTD

Lucknow • St Louis (USA) • Panama City (Panama) • London (UK) • Ahmedabad
Bengaluru • Chennai • Hyderabad • Kochi • Kolkata • Mumbai • Nagpur • New Delhi

Published by
Jitendar P Vij

Jaypee Brothers Medical Publishers (P) Ltd

Corporate Office
4838/24 Ansari Road, Daryaganj, **New Delhi** - 110002, India, Phone: +91-11-43574357, Fax: +91-11-43574314

Registered Office
B-3 EMCA House, 23/23B Ansari Road, Daryaganj, **New Delhi** - 110 002, India
Phones: +91-11-23272143, +91-11-23272703, +91-11-23282021
+91-11-23245672, Rel: +91-11-32558559, Fax: +91-11-23276490, +91-11-23245683
e-mail: jaypee@jaypeebrothers.com, Website: www.jaypeebrothers.com

Offices in India

- **Ahmedabad**, Phone: Rel: +91-79-32988717, e-mail: ahmedabad@jaypeebrothers.com
- **Bengaluru**, Phone: Rel: +91-80-32714073, e-mail: bangalore@jaypeebrothers.com
- **Chennai**, Phone: Rel: +91-44-32972089, e-mail: chennai@jaypeebrothers.com
- **Hyderabad**, Phone: Rel:+91-40-32940929, e-mail: hyderabad@jaypeebrothers.com
- **Kochi**, Phone: +91-484-2395740, e-mail: kochi@jaypeebrothers.com
- **Kolkata**, Phone: +91-33-22276415, e-mail: kolkata@jaypeebrothers.com
- **Lucknow**, Phone: +91-522-3040554, e-mail: lucknow@jaypeebrothers.com
- **Mumbai**, Phone: Rel: +91-22-32926896, e-mail: mumbai@jaypeebrothers.com
- **Nagpur**, Phone: Rel: +91-712-3245220, e-mail: nagpur@jaypeebrothers.com

Overseas Offices

- **North America Office, USA,** Ph: 001-636-6279734, e-mail: jaypee@jaypeebrothers.com, anjulav@jaypeebrothers.com
- **Central America Office, Panama City, Panama,** Ph: 001-507-317-0160, e-mail: cservice@jphmedical.com Website: www.jphmedical.com
- **Europe Office, UK,** Ph: +44 (0) 2031708910, e-mail: info@jpmedpub.com

Principles and Practice of Percutaneous Tracheostomy

© 2010, Jaypee Brothers Medical Publishers (P) Ltd.

This book has been published in good faith that the material provided by contributors is original. Every effort is made to ensure accuracy of material, but the publisher, printer and editor will not be held responsible for any inadvertent error (s). In case of any dispute, all legal matters are to be settled under Delhi jurisdiction only.

First Edition: **2010**

ISBN 978-81-8448-929-3

Typeset at JPBMP typesetting unit
Printed at   Replika Press Pvt. Ltd.

Contributors

Alan Šustić
Professor of Anaesthesiology and Intensive Care
Department of Anaesthesiology and Intensive Care
University Hospital Rijeka, T. Strizica 3, 51000
Rijeka, Croatia

Antonio Fantoni
Professor of Anestesia e Rianimazione
Department of Anaesthesia and Intensive Care
San Carlo Borromeo Hospital
Milan, Italy

Arturo Guarino
Department of Anaesthesia and Intensive Care
Medicine
Villa Scassi Hospital,
Geneva, Italy

Chandra Kant Pandey
Senior Consultant Anaesthetist
Sahara Hospital, Gomti Nagar
Lucknow, India

Christian Byhahn
Assistant Professor of Anesthesiology and
Intensive Care Medicine
Department of Anesthesiology
Intensive Care Medicine and Pain Control
J W Goethe-University Medical School
Theodor-Stern-Kai 7
D-60590 Frankfurt, Germany

Donata Ripamonti
Department of Anaesthesia and Intensive Care
San Carlo Borromeo Hospital
Milan, Italy

Giulio Frova
Professor and Director Emeritus
Department of Anesthesia and Intensive Care
Brescia Hospital
Brescia, Italy

Guido Merli
Department of Anaesthesia and
Intensive Care Medicine
Centro Cardiologico Monzino
Milano, Italy

Isha Tyagi
Professor of Otorhinolaryngology
Department of Neurosurgery
Sanjay Gandhi Postgraduate Institute
of Medical Sciences
Lucknow, India

Joseph L Nates
Associate Professor, Deputy Chair
Medical Director, Intensive Care Unit
Division of Anesthesiology and Critical Care
The University of Texas
MD Anderson Cancer Center
Houston, TX, USA

Massimiliano Sorbello
Anesthesia and Intensive Care
Policlinico University Hospital
Catania, Italy

Rudolph Puana
Assistant Professor
Critical Care Department, Division of
Anesthesiology and Critical Care
The University of Texas
MD Anderson Cancer Center
Houston, TX, USA

Sushil P Ambesh
Professor and Senior Consultant
Department of Anaesthesiology
Sanjay Gandhi Postgraduate Institute
of Medical Sciences
Lucknow, India

Foreword

The development of the percutaneous tracheostomy over the last two decades has revolutionized tracheostomy in critically ill patients. It has become an established procedure facilitating weaning from ventilatory support and shortening intensive care stay. Operative time is reduced and an operating theatre is not required. The risk of transferring a critically ill patient from ITU to theatre is also eliminated. It appears that long term sequelae are likely to be no more frequent than with surgical tracheostomy. There is no doubt that the development of the percutaneous tracheostomy will have proved to have been a major development in the management of critically ill patients.

In this context *Principles and Practice of Percutaneous Tracheostomy* written by professor Ambesh and co-authors provides a comprehensive overview of this important topic. This volume introduces us to the most recent developments in tracheostomy practice with a fascinating history of the origins of the tracheostomy. A detailed description of the various techniques is included, as is a catalogue of complications, contraindications and comparisons with surgical tracheostomy. The reader is taken through the practical procedures for different percutaneous tracheostomy techniques step by step with generous clear illustrations to guide him or her through the operation and avoiding potential difficulties and hazards. Many practical tips are included reflecting a wealth of underlying experience. Every aspect of this core topic in critical care medicine is covered.

As former colleagues of Professor Ambesh we are honored and delighted to write a foreword for this fine textbook, which not only teaches and instructs but also provides a fascinating insight into one of our most recently developed techniques in intensive care medicine. We have had first hand experience of the authors' skill and expertise, not just in the field of percutaneous tracheostomy but also his considerable clinical knowledge and abilities as an intensivist. It is with great pleasure that we recommend this outstanding textbook on the principles of percutaneous tracheostomy, which will prove to be an invaluable resource for all those involved in critical care.

TN Trotter and ES Lin
University Hospitals of Leicester, UK

Preface

Tracheostomy is one of the most commonly performed surgical procedures in intensive care unit patients and is indicated when airway protection, airway access or mechanical ventilation are needed for a prolonged period. Tracheostomy also facilitates weaning from the ventilator. Since its inception tracheostomy has remained in the domain of surgeons. Many a times the anesthesiologists or intensive care physicians looking after these patients get frustrated due to non-availability of the surgeon, operation room or encountered difficulties in shifting critically ill patients to operation room. This may have delayed timely formation of tracheostomy in needy patients. Anesthesiologists are supposed to be master in the art of airway management; however, dependency on surgeons to establish airway by surgical means gives a sense of incompleteness. With the advent of percutaneous dilatational tracheostomy (PDT), a bedside procedure, another much needed tool in airway management has been added in the armamentarium of anesthesiologists and intensive care physicians. Not only this, the PDT is gradually proving its superiority over surgical tracheostomy in many ways.

Over the last two decades surgical tracheostomy has largely been replaced by the PDT and more and more such procedures are being carried out worldwide. In early 1990s, when I was working as Anesthetic Registrar at Ulster Hospital, Dundonald, UK, my esteemed consultant Dr JM Murray, MD, FFARCSI taught me this procedure and I owe everything to him about this wonderful art of minimally invasive airway access. At that time, there were only two types of percutaneous tracheostomy kits: the Ciaglia's multiple dilators and Griggs guidewire dilating forceps. Presently, a number of PDT kits and techniques are available for clinical use and it is likely that further developments will take place in this field of airway access.

Advancement in readily available techniques of bedside percutaneous tracheostomy has carried respiratory therapy to a heightened level. Regrettably, many physicians remain ignorant of these clinically relevant advances and management of percutaneous tracheostomy and tracheostomized patients. Therefore, it is prudent to provide thorough knowledge of this important procedure to our trainees and colleagues who have been working in the field of anesthesia, intensive care unit, high dependency unit and pulmonary medicine. In this book I have tried to include all important and different PDT techniques available at present. There are various chapters written by guest authors' who have immensely contributed to the development and refinement of this novel technique. I sincerely hope that this comprehensive text on percutaneous tracheostomy alongwith relevant illustrations and pictures will be useful to the consultant anesthesiologist, intensivist, internist, chest physician, ENT surgeons and trainee residents.

Sushil P Ambesh

Acknowledgments

To my beloved wife Shashi and my two sons Paurush and Sahitya, without their constant encouragement, understanding and love this work could not have been possible.

To my loving parents IL Ambesh and Shanti Devi who taught me good social values, inspired me to become a doctor and have always been a constant source of inspiration.

To my revered teacher Dr JM Murray, MD, FFARCSI, Consultant in Anaesthesia and Intensive Care at Ulster Hospital, Dundonald, Belfast (UK) who taught me the art of minimally invasive airway management in early 1990s, when it was in its inception days.

My thanks are due to all the guest authors who have contributed many important chapters with high level of scientific and clinical knowledge. Their participation was fundamental to define the style of this publication. Special thanks with gratitude to Dr Matthias Gründling, Consultant Anesthetist and Intensivist at University of Greifswald, Germany who has provided a number of rare photographs from Archives of Anatomy, Greifswald.

My sincere thanks to Dr PK Singh, Professor and Head, Department of Anesthesiology, Sanjay Gandhi Postgraduate Institute of Medical Sciences, Lucknow (India) who has always encouraged and facilitated my scientific and academic endeavors.

Contents

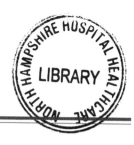
1. History of Tracheostomy and Evolution of Percutaneous Tracheostomy 1
   Sushil P Ambesh

2. Anatomy of the Larynx and Trachea 12
   Sushil P Ambesh

3. Indications, Advantages and Timing of Tracheostomy 18
   Sushil P Ambesh

4. Standard Surgical Tracheostomy 23
   Isha Tyagi, Sushil P Ambesh

5. Cricothyroidotomy 29
   Giulio Frova, Massimiliano Sorbello

6. Ciaglia's Techniques of Percutaneous Dilational Tracheostomy 39
   Rudolph Puana, Joseph L Nates, Sushil P Ambesh

7. Griggs' Technique of Percutaneous Dilational Tracheostomy 49
   Sushil P Ambesh

8. Frova's PercuTwist Percutaneous Dilational Tracheostomy 56
   Giulio Frova, Massimiliano Sorbello

9. Fantoni's Translaryngeal Tracheostomy Technique 65
   Donata Ripamonti

10. Balloon Facilitated Percutaneous Tracheostomy 80
    Christian Byhahn

11. Percutaneous Dilatational Tracheostomy with Ambesh T-Trach Kit 84
    Chandra Kant Pandey

12. Anesthetic and Technical Considerations for Percutaneous Tracheostomy 89
    Sushil P Ambesh

13. Complications and Contraindications of Percutaneous Tracheostomy 101
    Sushil P Ambesh

14. Percutaneous Dilational Tracheostomy in Special Situations 111
    Sushil P Ambesh

15. Percutaneous Tracheostomy versus Surgical Tracheostomy 116
    Arturo Guarino, Guido Merli

16. **How to Judge a Tracheostomy: A Reliable Method of Comparison of the Different Techniques** 124
Antonio Fantoni

17. **The Need to Compare Different Techniques of Tracheostomy in More Reliable Way** 130
Antonio Fantoni

18. **Care of Tracheostomy and Principles of Endotracheal Suctioning** 136
Sushil P Ambesh

19. **Ultrasound-guided Percutaneous Dilatational Tracheostomy** 149
Alan Šustić

20. **Tracheostomy Tubes, Decannulation and Speech** 155
Sushil P Ambesh

Index *163*

Abbreviations

ABP	Arterial blood pressure
COAD	Chronic obstructive airway disease
COPA	Cuffed oropharyngeal airway
CPAP	Continuous positive airway pressure
CT	Computed tomography
ECG	Electrocardiogram
ENT	Ear, nose and throat
ET tube	Endotracheal tube
EtCO$_2$	End-tidal carbondioxide
FG	French gauge
FiO$_2$	Fractional inspired oxygen
FOB	Fiberoptic bronchoscope
FRC	Functional residual capacity
GA	General anesthesia
GWDF	Guidewire delating forceps
HDU	High dependency unit
HME	Heat moisture exchanger
HMEF	Heat and moisture exchanging filter
ICP	Intracranial pressure
ICU	Intensive care unit
ID	Internal diameter
INR	International normalized ratio
IPPV	Intermittent positive pressure ventilation
LA	Local anesthesia
LMA	Laryngeal mask ventilation
min	Minute
PaCO$_2$	Partial pressure of carbon dioxide
PaO$_2$	Partial pressure of oxygen
PEEP	Positive end-expiratory pressure
PCT	Percutaneous tracheostomy
PDT	Percutaneous dilational tracheostomy
PLT	Platelets
s	Seconds
SaO$_2$	Arterial oxygen saturation
ST	Surgical tracheostomy
TIF	Tracheoinnominate artery fistula
TLT	Translaryngeal tracheostomy
TOF	Tracheoesophageal fistula
TT	Trachestomy tube
US	Ultrasound
WOB	Work of breathing

History of Tracheostomy and Evolution of Percutaneous Tracheostomy

Sushil P Ambesh

INTRODUCTION

Tracheostomy is one of the oldest surgical procedures described in the literature and refers to the formation of an opening or ostium into the anterior wall of trachea or the opening itself, whereas tracheotomy refers to the procedure to create an opening into the trachea (Fig. 1.1).[1] The term tracheostomy is used, by convention, for all these procedures and is considered synonymous with tracheotomy and is interchangeable. When done properly, it can save lives; yet the tracheotomy was not readily accepted by the medical community. The tracheotomy began as an emergency procedure, used to create an open airway for someone struggling for air. For most of its history, the tracheotomy was performed only as a last resort and mortality rates were very high.

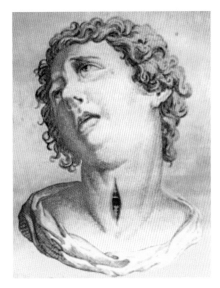

Fig. 1.1: Tracheostomy (*Courtesy:* Anatomy Library of University of Greifswald, Germany)

HISTORY OF TRACHEOSTOMY

One famous American whose life could have been saved by a tracheostomy was General George Washington, the first President of United States of America. At the end of the 18th century, however, the procedure was still considered too risky. In December 1799 Washington took his daily ride in heavy, wintry weather. He developed a sore throat and a malarial type of fever during the following days. He lay in his bed at Mount Vernon, Virginia, suffering from a septic sore throat and struggling for air (Fig. 1.2). Amongst the several physicians called to Washington's bedside was personal friend, Dr James Craik. Dr Craik and his colleagues diagnosed Washington with an "inflammatory quinsy", an inflammation of the throat accompanied by fever, swelling, and painful swallowing. Three physicians gathered around him and gave him sage

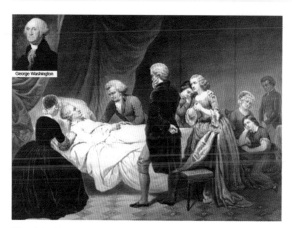

Fig. 1.2: George Washington lay in his bed at Mount Vernon, Virginia, suffering from a septic sore throat and struggling for air is attended by his friends and family members (*Courtesy:* Library of Congress)

tea with vinegar to gargle, but this increased the difficulty further and almost choked him. Elisha Cullen Dick, youngest amongst three physicians present, proposed a tracheotomy to help relieve the obstruction of the throat, but his suggestion was considered futile and irresponsible. He was vetoed by the other two physicians, who preferred more traditional treatment methods like bleeding by arteriotomy which was undertaken approximately four separate times equaling to a total loss of more than 2500 ml.[2] General Washington died that night. History buffs may recognize this story as the death of George Washington.[3] Modern day doctors now believe that Washington died from either a streptococcal infection of the throat, or a combination of shock from the loss of blood, asphyxia, and dehydration. One historian has stated that "whatever was the direct cause of General Washington's death, there can be little doubt that excessive bleeding reduced him to a low state and very much aggravated his disease." Had a tracheostomy been performed he could have been saved.

Only in the past century has the tracheotomy evolved into a safe and routine medical procedure. The tracheotomy is actually one of the oldest surgical procedures and a very ancient one. Tracheostomy has probably existed for more than 4000 years. *Rigveda*, an ancient sacred Hindu book referenced the tracheostomy dates back between 3000-2000 BC.[4] Egyptian wooden tablets depicts the surgical procedure of tracheostomy as early as 3000 BC.[5] One of the Egyptian tablets from the beginning of the first dynasty of King Aha was discovered to have engravings showing a seated person directing a pointed instrument towards the throat of another person (Fig. 1.3). Some people believe it human sacrifice but most experts believe that tablet depicts formation of a tracheostomy as human sacrifice was not practiced in ancient Egypt.

The history of surgical access to the airway is largely one of condemnation. This technique of slashing the throat to establish emergency airway access in order to save the life was known as "semi slaughter." During the Roman era, tracheostomies were performed using a large incision but with a warning to not to divide the whole of trachea as it could be fatal.[6]

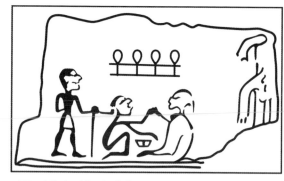

Fig. 1.3: A tablet depicting tracheotomy during the king Aha Dynasty

However, in largely hopeless cases of diphtheria, the opportunities tracheostomy offered for medical heroism ensured its place in the surgical armamentarium. Fabricius wrote in the 17th century, "This operation redounds to the honor of the physician and places him on a footing with the gods." Mcclelland had divided various phages of the evolution of tracheostomy into five periods: The period of legend: dating from 2000 BC to 1546; the period of fear: from 1546 to 1833 during which operation was performed only by a brave few, often at the risk of their reputation; the period of drama: from 1833 to 1932 during which the procedure was generally performed only in emergency situations as a life saving measure in patients with upper airway obstruction; the period of enthusiasm: from 1932 to 1965 during which the adage, 'if you think tracheostomy could be useful do it' became popular; and the period of rationalization; from 1965 to the present during which the relative merits of intubation versus tracheostomy were debated.[7] Various important dates in the evolution of tracheostomy are documented as follows:

- Approximately 400 BC: Hippocrates condemned tracheostomy, citing threat to carotid arteries.
- 100 BC: Asclepiades of Persia is credited as the first person to perform a tracheotomy in 100 BC. He described a tracheotomy incision for the treatment of upper airway obstruction due to pharyngeal inflammation. There is evidence that surgical incision into the trachea in an attempt to establish an artificial airway was performed by a Roman physician 124 years before the birth of Christ.
- Approximately 50 AD: Two physicians, Aretaeus and Galen, gave inflammation of the tonsils and larynx as indications for surgical tracheotomy. Aretaeus of Cappadocia warned against performing tracheotomy for infectious obstruction because of the risk of secondary wound infections.
- Approximately 100 AD: Antyllus described the first familiar tracheostomy: a horizontal incision between 2 tracheal rings to bypass upper airway obstruction. He also pointed out that tracheostomy would not ameliorate distal airway disease (e.g. bronchitis).
- 131 AD: Galen elucidated laryngeal and tracheal anatomy. He was the first to localize voice production to the larynx and to define laryngeal innervation. Additionally, he described the supralaryngeal contribution to respiration (e.g. warming, humidifying and filtering of inspired air).
- 400 AD: The *Talmud* advocated longitudinal incision in order to decrease bleeding. Caelius Aurelianus derided tracheostomy as a "senseless, frivolous, and even criminal invention of Asclepiades."
- 600 AD: The *Sushruta Samhita* contained routine acknowledgment of tracheostomy as accepted therapy in India.
- Approximately 600 AD: Dante pronounced it "a suitable punishment for a sinner in the depths of the Inferno."
- During the 11th century, Albucasis of Cordova successfully sutured the trachea of a servant who had attempted suicide by cutting her throat.
- 1546: The first record of a tracheostomy being performed in Europe was in the 16th century when Antonius Musa Brasavola (Fig. 1.4), an Italian physician performed a first documented tracheotomy and saved a patient who was suffering from laryngeal abscess and was in severe respiratory distress. The patient recovered from the procedure. Later, he published an account of tracheostomy for tonsillar obstruction. He was the first person known to actually perform the operation.

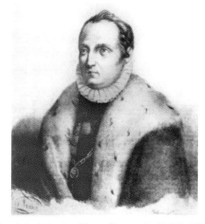

Fig. 1.4: Antonius Musa Brasavola (1490-1554)

- 1561-1636: As popularity of the operation increased, it was found that although asphyxia was immediately relieved, better long-term results were achieved if the stoma was kept patent for several days. Sanctorius was the first to use a trocar and cannula. He left the cannula in place for 3 days.
- 1550-1624: Habicot performed a series of 4 tracheostomies for obstructing foreign bodies.
- 1702-1743: George Martine developed the inner cannula.
- 1718: Lorenz Heister coined the term tracheotomy, which was previously known as laryngotomy or bronchotomy.
- 1739: Heister was the first to use the term tracheotomy and three decades later, Francis Home described an upper airway inflammation as Croup, and recommended tracheostomy to relieve obstructed airway.
- 1800-1900: Before 1800 only 50 life-saving tracheotomies had been described in the literature (Fig. 1.5). In 1805 Viq d'Azur described cricothyrotomy. A major interest in tracheostomy developed after Napoleon Bonaparte's nephew died of diphtheria in 1807.

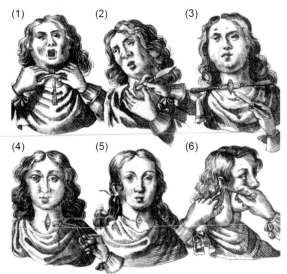

Fig. 1.5: First five photographs (1666) showing the steps of tracheostomy (*Courtesy:* Health Sciences Libraries, University of Washington)

Research into the technique got a boost with resurrection of some of the old instruments. During the diphtheria epidemic in France in 1825, tracheostomies gained further recognition. Improvements followed: 1833: Trousseau reported 200 patients with diphtheria treated with tracheostomy. In 1852, Bourdillat developed a primitive pilot tube; in 1869 Durham introduced the famous lobster-tail tube; and in 1880 the first pediatric tracheostomy tube was introduced by Parker. Later, introduction of endotracheal intubation in the early 20th century and high mortality rate associated with tracheostomy led to sharp decline in the formation of tracheostomy procedure. During and before this period some very interesting surgical tools were developed to form rapid tracheal stoma and some of these are shown in Figs 1.6 and 1.7.

- 1909: Chevalier Jackson (Fig. 1.8) standardized the technique of surgical tracheostomy and published the operative details of this procedure.[8] He codified the indications and techniques for modern tracheostomy and warned of complications of high tracheostomy and cricothyroidotomy. Since then it became an important part of the surgeon's armamentarium.
- 1932: Wilson advocated prophylactic tracheostomy in patients with poliomyelitis to facilitate the removal of secretions and to prevent pulmonary infections.

EVOLUTION OF CUFFED TRACHEOSTOMY TUBE

From Mid 1800s to 1970 metallic tracheostomy tubes were in clinical practice (Fig. 1.9). These tubes were associated with high rate of tracheal complications and aspiration pneumonia. Tredenlenburg, in 1969, first proposed the incorporation of cuff in a tracheostomy tube. However, it was not until the development of positive pressure ventilation (IPPV) that required cuffed tracheostomy tube. Until mid 1970s, the

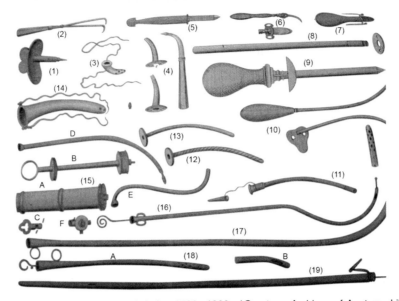

Fig. 1.6: Tracheostomy tools used during 1700s-1900s (*Courtesy:* Archives of Anatomy Library, University of Greifswald, Germany)

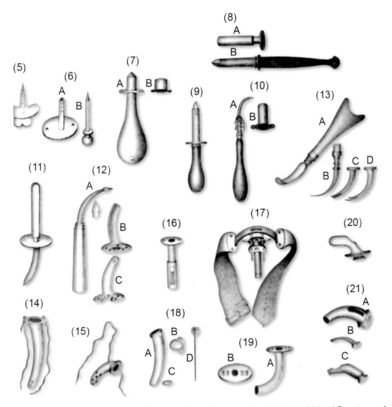

Fig. 1.7: Some more surgical tools used to perform tracheostomy during 1700s-1900s (*Courtesy:* Archives of Anatomy Library, University of Greifswald, Germany)

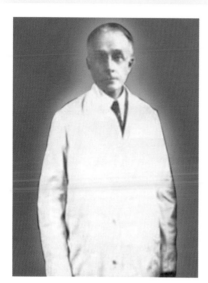

Fig. 1.8: Chevalier Q Jackson (1865-1958) who described step by step account of surgical tracheostomy

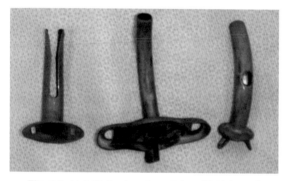

Fig. 1.9: Metallic tracheostomy tube with plain and fenestrated inner cannulas

cuffs of endotracheal as well as the tracheostomy tubes were low-volume, high-pressure and were indicated for short-term use during the operative procedures under general anesthesia. In 1960s, a number of tracheal mucosal injuries were reported with these tubes, if used for longer duration. This led to the development of high-volume, low-pressure cuffs in polyvinyl chloride or silicone tubes (Fig. 1.10). These cuffs when inflated provide larger surface area for contact with the trachea, therefore minimizing tracheal mucosa ischemia and destruction.

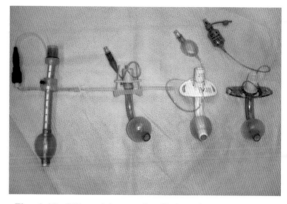

Fig. 1.10: Different types of cuffed tracheostomy tubes

In the last three decades, while emergency tracheostomy has become a rarity, elective tracheostomy has become more common due to the increasing awareness of complications caused by prolonged translaryngeal intubation for long-term airway access.

EVOLUTION OF PERCUTANEOUS TRACHEOSTOMY

With the passage of time the extensive surgical procedures are being replaced with minimally invasive or keyhole surgical procedure and the tracheostomy cannot remain an exception. Historically, various devices were available for rapid formation of tracheostomy through percutaneous approach; however, such devices were inherently unsafe due to their design and never achieved widespread usage. Since late 1980s a number of percutaneous tracheostomy devices have been introduced in clinical practice with excellent results. A review of historical aspects of percutaneous tracheostomy is presented below:

Seldinger (1953) introduced the technique of guide wire needle replacement in percutaneous arterial catheterization; and soon after the technique became popular as Seldinger technique.[9] This technique has been adapted to various procedures, including percutaneous tracheostomy.

Shelden (1957) was first to introduce percutaneous tracheotomy in an attempt to reduce the incidence of complications that followed open surgical tracheostomy and to obviate the need to move potentially unstable intensive care patients to the operating theater. Shelden and colleagues gained airway access with a slotted needle then that was used to guide a cutting trocar into the trachea (Fig. 1.11).[10] Unfortunately, the method caused multiple complications; and fatalities were reported secondary to the trocar's laceration of vital structures adjacent to the airway.

Toye and Weinstein (1969) used a tapered straight dilator that was advanced into the tracheal airway over a guide catheter. This tapered dilator had a recessed blade that was designed to cut tissue as the dilator was forced into the trachea over a guiding catheter.[11] However, this device too was associated with complications like peritracheal insertion, tracheal injuries, esophageal perforation and hemorrhage; and is therefore now obsolete.

Ciaglia P (1985) thoracic surgeon ((Fig. 1.12), described a technique that relies on progressive blunt dilatation of a small initial tracheal aperture created by a needle using series of graduated dilators over a guide wire that had been inserted into the

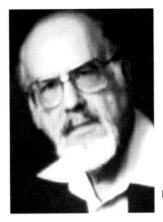

Fig. 1.12: Pasquale (Pat) Ciaglia (1912-2000)

trachea.[12] A formal tracheostomy tube is passed into the trachea over an appropriately sized dilator. He modified percutaneous nephrostomy set to facilitate percutaneous tracheostomy in a series of 26 patients. As early results of percutaneous tracheostomy were favorably comparable with surgical tracheostomy, by 1990 the technique became quite popular. The kit is being manufactured by Cook Critical Care, Bloomington, IN, USA (Fig. 1.13) Ciaglia is regarded as father of modern bedside percutaneous tracheostomy and whose approach rejuvenated the interest in the art and clinical utility of tracheostomy.

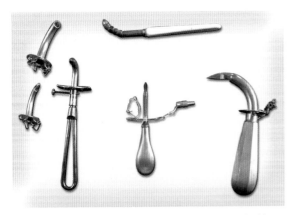

Fig. 1.11: Cutting trocar and cannula (*Courtesy:* Archives of Anatomy Library of University of Greifswald, Germany)

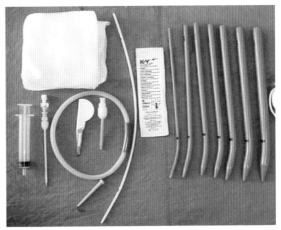

Fig. 1.13: Ciaglia's percutaneous dilatational tracheostomy introducer set (Cook Inc, Bloomington, IN, USA)

Schachner A (1989) developed a kit (Rapitrach, Fresenius) that consisted of a cutting edged dilating forceps (Fig. 1.14) with a beveled metal conus designed to advance forcibly over a guide wire and opened, allowing a tracheostomy tube to be inserted between the open jaws of the device.[13] Rapitrach kit, as the name suggests, was originally designed for emergency use to gain airway access to trachea through percutaneous approach but the kit was associated with a number of posterior tracheal wall injury reports and even death.

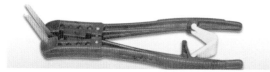

Fig. 1.14: Rapitrach dilating forceps (Surgitech, Sydney, Australia)

Griggs WM (1990) reported a guide wire dilating forceps (GWDF) marketed by Portex, Hythe Kent, UK (Fig. 1.15).[14] The device is like a pair of modified Kelly's forceps but does not have a cutting edge of the Rapitrach. The GWDF is passed into the trachea after initial dilation over a guide wire. Griggs forceps is quite popular in European countries and Australia.

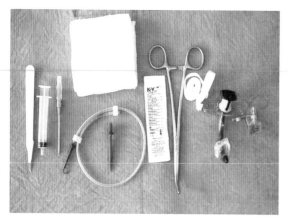

Fig. 1.15: Griggs guide wire dilating forceps kit with tracheostomy tube (SIMS Portex Ltd, Hythe, Kent, UK)

Fantoni A (1993) described a technique of tracheostomy through translaryngeal approach whose main feature was the passage of a dilator as well as the tracheostomy tube from inside of the trachea to the outside of the neck (an in and out technique).[15] The tracheostomy tube is pulled from inside the trachea to the outside and rotated. The initial version of the kit was later modified in 1997 (Mallinckrodt, Europe) (Fig. 1.16).[16]

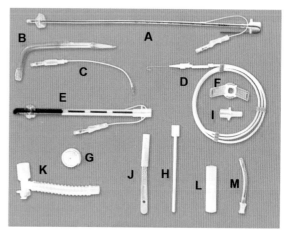

Fig. 1.16: Fantoni's translaryngeal tracheostomy kit (Mallinckrodt Medical GmbH, Hennef, Germany)

Ciaglia P (1999) developed a modification of his own technique wherein a series of dilators was replaced with a single, sharply tapered dilator with a hydrophilic coating that looks like Rhino's horn and therefore appropriately named Blue Rhino (Cook Critical Care, Bloomington, IN, USA) (Fig. 1.17). The device permits formation of tracheal stoma in one step for insertion of a tracheostomy tube using Seldinger guide wire technique.

Ciaglia P (2000) shortly before his death at the age of 88 years, came up with an idea of balloon facilitated percutaneous tracheostomy (BFPT). His preliminary vision was translated into the reality by Michael Zgoda, a pulmonologist at the University of Kentucky (USA) and published his experience using this kit in 2003 (Fig. 1.18).[17]

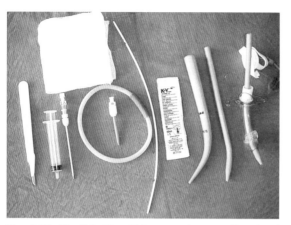

Fig. 1.17: Ciaglia's Blue Rhino percutaneous dilatational tracheostomy introducer set (Cook Critical Care, Bloomington, IN, USA)

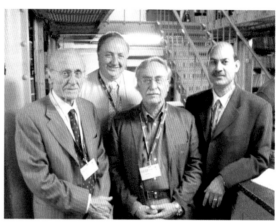

Fig. 1.19: (Left to Right): A Fantoni, WM Griggs, G Frova and SP Ambesh. 1st International Symposium "Tracheostomy-Past and Present" at University of Greifswald, Germany (11-13 May 2006)

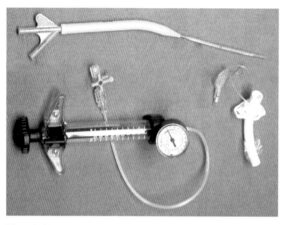

Fig. 1.18: Ciaglia's Blue Dolphin Balloon Dilatation percutaneous tracheostomy introducer (Cook Critical care, Bloomington, IN, USA)

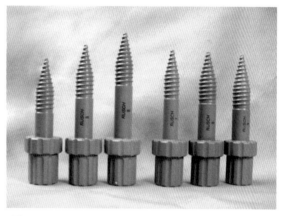

Fig. 1.20: Different sizes of Frova's PercuTwist dilators (Ruüsch, Kernen, Germany)

Frova G (2002) Professor of Anesthesia and Intensive Care at Brescia Hospital, Italy (Fig. 1.19) developed a screw like device (PercuTwist[®], Rüsch) that utilizes a self-tapering screw dilator to form tracheal stoma over the guide wire.[18] The screw like dilator (Fig. 1.20) is claimed to offer more controlled dilation of the trachea without causing anterior tracheal wall compression.

Ambesh SP (2005) Professor of Anesthesiology at Sanjay Gandhi Postgraduate Institute of Medical Sciences, Lucknow (India) (Fig. 1.19) introduced

a modification to Ciaglia Blue Rhino by developing a T-shaped tracheal dilator "T-Trach" (formerly known as T-Dagger). Unlike Ciaglia's rounded dilator, the shaft of T-Trach is elliptical in shape with tapered edges, and has a number of oval holes (Fig. 1.21).[19] Like other techniques of PDT, T-Trach too utilizes Seldinger guide wire technique. As this is a very recent addition to the range of percutaneous tracheostomy kits, only few studies are available at the moment. However, it has been claimed that the T-trach has a potential of

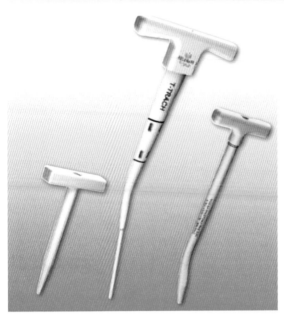

Fig. 1.21: Ambesh's T-Trach percutaneous tracheostomy introducer (Eastern Medikit Limited, Delhi, India)

minimizing tracheal injuries and cartilaginous rings fracture while causing creation of tracheal stoma between the two tracheal rings, in one step.

A large number of studies have been conducted with various commercially available PDT kits. Many authors are proponents of the technique for the formation of elective tracheostomy in intensive care unit patients for long-term ventilation, isolation of airway and weaning from ventilator.[20] Other authors have reported no significant superiority of PDT over traditional surgical tracheostomy. Recently, Paw and Turner in their survey reported that percutaneous tracheostomy is being performed in 75% of intensive care units of England and Wales and has almost replaced the surgical tracheostomy. The most commonly used percutaneous tracheostomy kit was Ciaglia's multiple serial dilators (46.6%) followed by Ciaglia's Blue Rhino kit (31.3%).[21] However, irrespective of the techniques used the most common thing is the use of guide wire. The most important and major modification to the technique is the increasing use

of the fiberoptic bronchoscope to visualize the placement of tracheal puncture needle, the guide wire and the tracheostomy tube. A detailed description on commonly used percutaneous tracheostomy kits and the techniques is presented in the succeeding chapters of the book.

REFERENCES

1. Hensyl WR, (Ed). Stedman's medical dictionary. 25th ed. Baltimore, MD: Williams and Wilkins 1990;1616.
2. Cheatham ML. The death of George Washington: An end to the controversy? Am Surg 2008;74(8): 770-4.
3. Morens DM. Death of a president. New Eng J Med 1999;341:1845-9.
4. Frost EAM. Tracing the tracheostomy. Ann Otol Rhinol Laryngol 1976;85:618-24.
5. Pahor AI. Ear, nose and throat in Ancient Egypt. J Laryngol Otol 1992;106:773-9.
6. Van Heurn LWE, Brink PRG. The history of percutaneous tracheotomy. J Laryngol Otol 1996;110: 723-6.
7. Mcclelland MA. Tracheostomy: Its management and alternatives. Proceedings of the Royal Society of Medicine 1972;65:401-3.
8. Jackson C. Tracheostomy. Laryngoscope 1909;19: 285-90.
9. Seldinger SI. Catheter replacement of the needle in percutaneous arteriography. Acta Radiol 1953;39: 368-76.
10. Sheldon CH, Pudenz RH, Freshwater DB, Crue BL. A new method for tracheotomy. J Neurosurg 1957;12: 428-31.
11. Toye FJ, Weinstein JD. A percutaneous tracheostomy device. Surgery 1969;65:384-9.
12. Ciaglia P, Firsching R, Syniec C. Elective percutaneous dilatational tracheostomy: A new simple bedside procedure; preliminary report. Chest 1985;87:715-9.
13. Schachner A, Ovil Y, Sidi J, Rogev M, Heilbronn Y, Levy MJ. Percutaneous tracheostomy: A new method. Crit Care Med 1989;17:1052-6.
14. Griggs WM, Worthley LI, Gilligan JE, Thomas PD, Myburg JA. A simple percutaneous tracheostomy technique. Surg Gynaecol Obstet 1990;170:543-5.
15. Fantoni A. Translaryngeal tracheostomy. In:Gullo A (Ed). API-CE Trieste 1993;459-5.
16. Fantoni A, Ripamonti D. A non-derivative, non-surgical tracheostomy: The translaryngeal method. Intens Care Med 1997;23:386-92.

17. Zgoda M, Berger R. Balloon facilitated percutaneous tracheostomy tube placement: A novel technique. Chest 2003;124:130S-1S.

18. Frova G, Quintel M. A new simple method of percutaneous tracheostomy: Controlled rotating dilation. Intens Care Med 2002;28:299-303.

19. Ambesh SP, Tripathi M, Pandey CK, Pant KC, Singh PK. Clinical evaluation of the 'T-Dagger™': A new bedside percutaneous dilational tracheostomy device. Anaesthesia 2005;60:708-11.

20. Kearney PA, et al. A single-center 8-year experience with percutaneous dilational tracheostomy. Ann Surg 2000;231:701.

21. Paw HGW, Turner S. The current state of percutaneous tracheostomy in intensive care: A postal survey. Clin Intens Care 2002;13:95-101.

Chapter 2

Anatomy of the Larynx and Trachea

Sushil P Ambesh

THE LARYNX

The larynx is a space that communicates above with the laryngeal part of the pharynx, and below with the trachea. Apart from being a respiratory passage the larynx is an organ of phonation, and has a sphincteric mechanism. Near the middle of the larynx there is a pair of vocal folds (one right and one left) that project into the laryngeal cavity. Between these folds there is an interval called the rima-glottidis. The rima is fairly wide in ordinary breathing. When we wish to speak the two vocal cords come close together narrowing the rima-glottidis. Expired air passing through the narrow gap causes the vocal folds to vibrate resulting in the production of sound. It projects ventrally between the great vessels of the neck, and is covered anteriorly by the skin, fasciae and depressor muscles of the hyoid bone. Above, it opens into the laryngeal part of the pharynx and below it is continuous with trachea. It lays opposite the third, fourth, fifth and sixth cervical vertebrae in adult male while it is situated little higher in child and adult female. In Caucasian adults its length varies from 36 mm to 42 mm, transverse diameter from 41 mm to 43 mm and anteroposterior diameter from 26 mm to 36 mm. Larynx is constructed mainly from cartilages, ligaments and muscles. The skeletal framework of larynx is composed of nine cartilages: three large unpaired (single) cartilages and three small paired cartilages. The three large unpaired cartilages are the epiglottis, the thyroid, and the cricoid. The three paired cartilages are the arytenoids, cuneiforms, and the corniculates.

The **thyroid cartilage** is the largest cartilage of the larynx. It consists of the two quadrilateral laminae, the caudal parts of the anterior borders of which are fused at an angle (about 90° in male and about 120° in female) in the median plane to form a subcutaneous projection named Adam's apple. The cephalic portion of the laminae has an anterior gap and forms a V-shaped notch that is known as superior thyroid notch (Figs 2.1 and 2.2). The caudal parts of the anterior borders of the right and left laminae fuse and form a median projection called the laryngeal prominence. The posterior margins of the laminae are prolonged upwards to form a projection called the superior cornu; and downwards to form a smaller projection called the inferior cornu. The medial side of each inferior cornu articulates with the corresponding lateral aspect of the cricoid cartilage. The lateral surface of each lamina is marked by an oblique line that runs downwards and forwards. At its upper and lower ends the oblique line ends in projections called superior and inferior tubercles, respectively.

The cricoid is a signet ring like circumferential cartilage. It is smaller, but thicker and stronger than thyroid cartilage and forms the caudal part of the anterior and lateral walls and most of the posterior wall of the larynx. This is the narrowest part of the larynx in a child and consequently determines the size of the tracheal tube. Naturally, any edema of the mucosal surface can reduce the airway diameter. considerably. In an adult larynx the narrowest part is at the level of the vocal cords. Application of pressure on cricoid cartilage occludes the esophageal lumen and is a very important maneuver to prevent regurgitation and aspiration of gastric contents during induction of general anesthesia in patients with full stomach. This maneuver is known as Sellick's maneuver.[1] The cricothyroid ligament or membrane stretches between the thyroid and cricoid cartilages (Figs 2.1 and 2.2). The cricothyroid muscle arises from the anterior surface of the cricoid and travels superiorly, posteriorly, and laterally to attach laterally to the surface of the thyroid cartilage. This muscle rotates the thyroid anteriorly and lengthens the vocal cords. The vocalis muscles arise from the inner surface of the thyroid

cartilage in the midline and pass superiorly and posteriorly to attach to the length of the vocal cords. They shorten the cords and vary the tension on the cords. These two pairs of muscles and the cords are vulnerable to injury during cricothyrotomy.

The Epiglottis cartilage is tongue shaped, having a broad upper part and a narrow lower end. It is attached inferiorly to the posterior aspect of the thyroid cartilage by the thyroepiglottic ligament. The anterior surface is free and usually visualized at laryngoscopy. The posterior surface of the epiglottis is attached to the hyoid bone.

The arytenoids cartilages are pyramidal in shape and are placed on the superior and lateral border of the laminae of the cricoid cartilage. The lateral and posterior cricoarytenoid muscles are inserted into two of the three corners of the pyramidal base. The third corner provides the attachment for the vocal ligament. The arytenoids cartilage articulates with the cricoid cartilage and forms a synovial joint. The corniculate and cuneiform cartilages are very small and are of little importance in the structure of the larynx in terms of applied anatomy for tracheostomy procedures.

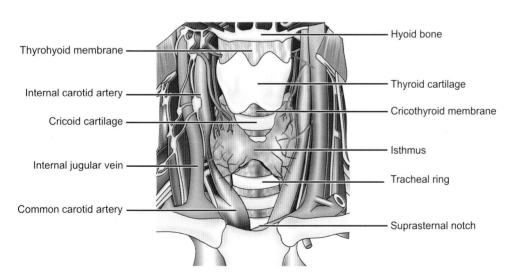

Fig. 2.1: Anterior view of the larynx and trachea with neighboring structures

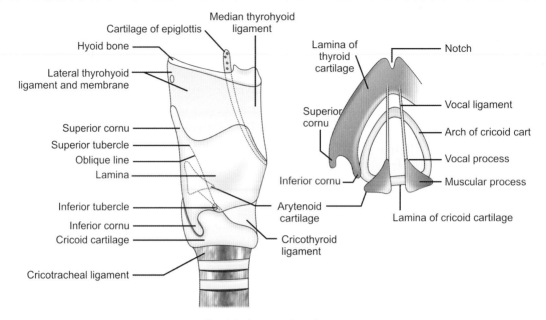

Fig. 2.2: Laryngeal cartilages

THE LARYNGEAL LIGAMENTS

The thyrohyoid membrane is one of the three extrinsic ligaments and runs between the hyoid bone and the upper border of the thyroid cartilage. Medially, it is quite dense and forms the median thyrohyoid ligament. Posteriorly, the ligament stretches from the greater horn of the hyoid to the upper horn of the thyroid cartilage. Laterally, these attachments are very dense and form the lateral thyrohyoid ligaments.

The hyoid bone is supported by the hypoglossus and median constrictor muscles. The superior laryngeal blood vessels and internal branch of superior laryngeal nerve pass through this membrane to supply the larynx above the vocal cords. Superiorly, fibrous tissue connects the base of the epiglottis to the arytenoids cartilages and this free upper surface is termed the aryepiglottic fold. Inferiorly, this fibrous tissue thickens to form the vestibular ligament. The mucous membranes run from the medial edge of the aryepiglottic fold down over these fibrous connections and terminate around the vestibular ligament to form the false cords. Below the false cords there is a thin horizontal recess called the sinus of the larynx. Another membrane, termed cricovocal membrane, is attached inferiorly to the cricoid cartilage and runs upwards and forwards to be attached anteriorly to the thyroid cartilage and posteriorly to the vocal process of the arytenoids cartilage. The free surface, which is also the lower border of the sinus of the larynx, forms the vocal ligament. The vocal ligaments are covered by mucous membranes and become the vocal cords. The cricovocal membrane is thickened in front and is termed the median cricothyroid ligament. Laterally, it is called lateral cricothyroid ligament.

LARYNGEAL MUSCLES

The laryngeal muscles are divided into two groups: the extrinsic and intrinsic. The extrinsic muscles attach the larynx to nearby structures and are responsible for elevation and depression of the larynx. The intrinsic muscles are important for deglutition and phonation. The posterior cricoarytenoid muscle is the only abductor of the vocal cords.

RELATIONS OF LARYNX

Anteriorly, the larynx is related to the superficial fascia and the skin of the neck. The thyroid and cricoid cartilages can be palpated easily through the skin and are important landmarks to identify cricothyroid membrane while performing cricothyrotomy during emergency airway management. The superior laryngeal nerves lie between superior cornu of thyroid cartilage and greater horn of hyoid bone on both sides. This nerve may be blocked with 2% lignocaine for an awake endotracheal intubation.

VASCULAR AND NERVE SUPPLY

The larynx derives its blood supply from laryngeal branches of the superior and inferior thyroid arteries (Fig. 2.1). The veins accompanying the superior laryngeal artery join the superior thyroid vein which opens into the internal jugular vein; those accompanying the inferior laryngeal artery join the inferior thyroid vein, which opens into the left brachiocephalic vein.

The larynx is supplied by (i) superior laryngeal nerve that divides into two external and internal branches and (ii) the recurrent laryngeal nerves. The external branch of superior laryngeal nerve supplies the cricothyroid muscle while the internal branch after piercing the thyrohyoid membrane provide the sensory supply down to the vocal cords. The recurrent laryngeal nerves from left and right sides run upwards in the neck in the groove between the esophagus and trachea. They provide sensory fibers below the vocal cords and supply all of the intrinsic muscles of the larynx except the cricothyroid. In addition, it supplies sensory branches to the mucous membrane of the larynx below the vocal cords. The damage to any of these

main nerves may present clinically as a hoarse voice and render the larynx incompetent with a potential for aspiration. In the event of bilateral recurrent laryngeal nerve damage, the action of the superior laryngeal nerve remains unopposed. This results in abduction of vocal cords and acute airway obstruction due to bilateral contraction of cricothyroid muscle. These patients generally require tracheostomy. Complete paralysis of both, the recurrent laryngeal and superior laryngeal nerves, bring the vocal cords in midway position (cadaveric position); however, this is not fraught with difficulty in breathing.

THE TRACHEA

The trachea is a cartilaginous membranous tubular structure that lies mainly on the front of the neck more or less in the median plane. The upper end of trachea is continuous with the lower end of the larynx (Fig. 2.3). The junction lies opposite the lower part of the body of sixth cervical vertebra and cricoid cartilage. It terminates at the level of 4th thoracic vertebra where it divides into left and right bronchi.[2]

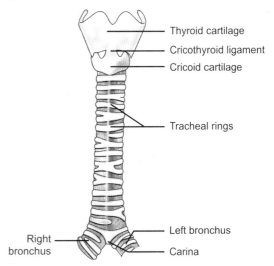

Fig. 2.3: Trachea is formed with 16-20 C-shaped cartilages

In the normal anatomical position, in an adult the length of the trachea ranges from 10–14 cm, but varies with age, sex and race; approximately 50% is above and 50% is below the suprasternal notch. It extends from the larynx through the neck to the thorax, where it terminates at the carina, dividing into the right and left main stem bronchi, one for each lung. It is not a cylindrical structure, being flattened posteriorly. Its external diameter from side to side is about 1.5 to 2.5 cm in adults and root of the index finger gives a rough idea about the tracheal diameter. The tracheal architecture consists of 16-20 horizontal 'C' shaped cartilages which are joined posteriorly by the trachealis muscles. Vertically, these cartilages are joined to each other by fibro-elastic tissue and give an appearance similar to that of tyres piled one on top of the other. The first and last tracheal cartilages differ from the others. The first cartilage is broader than the rest, and often deviated at one end that is connected with the cricotracheal ligament with the lower border of cricoid cartilage. The last cartilage is thick and broad in the middle, where its lower border is prolonged into a triangular hook-shaped process which curves downwards and backwards between the two bronchi forming a ridge called carina. These anterior cartilages provide the rigidity necessary to maintain patency of the tube. Each of the cartilages is enclosed in a perichondrium, which is continuous with a sheet of dense irregular connective tissue forming a fibrous membrane between adjacent hoops of cartilage and at the posterior aspect of the trachea where the cartilage is incomplete. The trachea is very mobile and can extend and shorten during deep inspiration and expiration. When the neck is extended a larger portion of the trachea becomes extrathoracic and when flexed larger portion becomes intrathoracic. On deep inspiration the carina may descend up to the level of 6th thoracic vertebra. The tracheal wall consists of four layers: mucosa, submucosa, cartilage, and adventitia. The inner layer, the mucosa, has ciliated pseudo-stratified columnar epithelium with goblet cells. Mucus excreted from the goblet cells helps trap inhaled particles of dust and the cilia sweep it upward into the laryngopharynx where it can be swallowed or coughed out. The submucosa is loose connective tissue containing glands that secrete mucus.

Relations of Trachea

Although the trachea is a midline structure in the neck, the lower aspect is displaced to the right by the aortic arch. The cervical part of the trachea is covered anteriorly with the skin and the superficial and deep fasciae. The isthmus of the thyroid runs across the trachea at the level of the 7th cervical vertebra and 2nd, 3rd and 4th rings of the trachea (Figs 2.1 and 2.4). Either side of the isthmus are the thyroid lobes. Immediately above the isthmus there is an anastomosing vessel that connects two superior thyroid arteries. Below, the isthmus it is related, in front, to the pretracheal fascia, the inferior thyroid veins, the remains of the thymus and the arteria thyroidea ima. Posteriorly, there lies esophagus in close relationship while the recurrent laryngeal nerves are found running laterally in both tracheoesophageal grooves. At the suprasternal notch the trachea enters the superior mediastinum. The innominate artery, or brachiocephalic trunk, crosses from left to right anterior to the trachea at the superior thoracic inlet and lies just beneath the sternum. Laterally on the right side, the trachea has a close relationship with the mediastinal pleura, the azygos vein and the vagus nerve. On the left side, the aortic arch and the major left sided arteries come between the trachea and pleura.[3] There may be aberrant position of the blood vessels. Hatfield and Bodenham[4] found that two of their 30 patients had carotid arteries in the immediate paratracheal position, whilst another two had prominent brachiocephalic arteries. Half of the patients had anterior jugular veins and eight were near the midline at considerable risk, necessitating appropriate 'safety measures'.

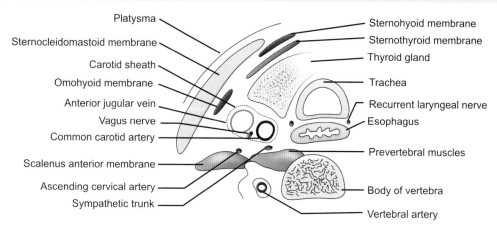

Fig. 2.4: Structures in relations to trachea

The recurrent laryngeal nerves and inferior thyroid veins that travel in the tracheoesophageal groove are paratracheal structures vulnerable to injury if dissection strays from the midline. The great vessels (i.e. carotid arteries, internal jugular veins) could be damaged should dissection go far a field. This is a real risk in obese or pediatric patients.

VASCULAR AND NERVE SUPPLY

The trachea obtains its blood supply mainly from the inferior thyroid arteries. Its thoracic end is supplied by the bronchial arteries, which give off branches ascending to anastomose with the inferior thyroid arteries. The veins drain into the inferior thyroid venous plexus. The sensory innervation of trachea and vocal cords is from the recurrent laryngeal branches of the vagus nerve which also carry sympathetic nerve endings from the middle cervical ganglion. This can be blocked by instillation of 2% lignocaine (4 ml) puncturing cricothyroid membrane. The sensory innervation of skin over the trachea comes from the roots C2-C4 of cervical plexus that can be blocked by subcutaneous infiltration with 2% lignocaine (10 ml).

REFERENCES

1. Sellick BA. Cricoid pressure to control regurgitation of stomach contents during induction of anaesthesia. Lancet 1961;2:404-6.
2. Warwick R, Williams PL. Gray's Anatomy 35th Edition, Longman 1973.
3. Difficulties in tracheal intubation. (Eds) Latto IP and Rosen M. Publ. Bailliere Tindall (1st edn. 1985).
4. Hatfield A, Bodenham A. Portable ultrasonic scanning of the anterior neck before percutaneous dilatational tracheostomy. Anaesthesia 1999;54:660-3.

Indications, Advantages and Timing of Tracheostomy

Sushil P Ambesh

Since the earliest beginning of critical care medicine, tracheostomy has been a valuable procedure to provide airway access for patients with acute airway problems. For the last five decades, the tracheostomy is most often performed as an elective procedure to provide airway access for critically ill patients who require prolonged artificial respiratory support.[1] In1960s to mid 1970s, the rigid design of endotracheal tube with low volume high pressure cuff, that has been associated with laryngotracheal complications, promoted the early placement of tracheostomies, within 3 days of respiratory failure, for patients requiring long-term ventilatory support. Following the introduction of modern endotracheal tubes in late 1970s and early 1980s, the use of tracheostomy declined as these endotracheal tubes favored prolonged translaryngeal intubation as compared to relatively higher incidence of complications associated to tracheostomy.[2]

The 1989, Association of Critical Care and Chest Physicians (ACCP) Consensus Conference on Artificial Airways in patients receiving mechanical ventilation recommended tracheostomy for patients whose anticipated need for artificial airway is more than 21 days.[3] It also recommended that the decision to convert a translaryngeal intubation to a tracheostomy be made as early as possible during the course of management of the patient to minimize the duration of translaryngeal intubation. Conversion from translaryngeal intubation to tracheostomy may facilitate nursing care, bronchial toilet, feeding, and mobility and promote early return of speech. Tracheostomy may facilitate the weaning process in patients with limited ventilatory capacity by reducing the airway resistance and work of breathing and thereby potentially reducing intensive care unit (ICU) stay.[4]

In patients requiring emergency airway for artificial ventilation or isolation of airway the translaryngeal intubation under general anesthesia and relaxation remains the first choice as it can be done with not much time wasting. However, the translaryngeal tube cannot be kept for a long time in critically sick patients as it may be associated with various complications. The complications of prolonged translaryngeal intubations are well recognized.

COMPLICATIONS OF PROLONGED TRANSLARYNGEAL INTUBATION

- Patient discomfort
- Poor or inadequate oropharyngeal hygiene, mucosal ulcers and oral thrush
- Requirement of sedation to tolerate the translaryngeal tube
- Increased risk of laryngeal injury

- Inadvertent extubation
- Ulcerations of nares or lips, pharynx and larynx (Fig. 3.1)
- Posterior glottic and subglottic stenosis
- Vocal cord lacerations or paralysis
- Sinusitis
- Posterior glottic and subglottic stenosis
- Damage to intrinsic muscle
- Vocal cord fixation from fibrosis of the crico-arytenoid joint
- Dislocation or subluxation of the arytenoids cartilages
- Tracheal injuries (tracheomalacia, tracheal dilatation, and tracheal stenosis)
- Aspiration pneumonia

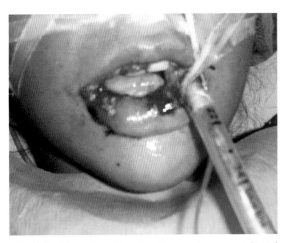

Fig. 3.1: Ulceration, bleeding lips and poor orodental hygiene in a patient with oral endotracheal tube for 10 days

Formation of tracheostomy may be necessary in patients with upper airway obstruction caused by trauma, infection, burns, malignancy, laryngeal and subcricoid stenosis. Percutaneous tracheostomy is not preferred in upper airway obstruction and is relatively contraindicated.

INDICATIONS FOR TRACHEOSTOMY

Tracheostomy becomes a consideration in patients who have upper airway obstruction or in intubated, critically ill patients in whom successful weaning and extubation cannot be achieved after a period of mechanical ventilation. Various indications of tracheostomy are as follows:[5-9]

- To relieve upper airway obstruction
  - Foreign body
  - Trauma
  - Acute infection–acute epiglottitis, diphtheria, retropharyngeal abscess
  - Glottic edema
  - Bilateral abductor paralysis of the vocal cords
  - Tumors of the larynx
  - Congenital web or atresia
  - Severe sleep apnea not amendable to continuous positive airway pressure (CPAP) devices or other, less invasive surgery
- To improve respiratory function and to provide prolonged mechanical ventilation
    Bronchopneumonia refractory to treatment
  - Severe chronic obstructive pulmonary disease
  - Chronic bronchitis and emphysema
  - Acute respiratory distress syndrome
  - Chest injury and flail chest
  - Severe brain injury
  - Multiple organ system dysfunction
  - Tetanus
- Respiratory paralysis
  - Unconscious patients, head injury, intracranial bleed
  - Bulbar poliomyelitis
  - Guillain-Barre syndrome, myasthenia gravis and other neurological disorders
- Airway access for secretions removal and tracheobronchial toilette
  - Inadequate cough due to chronic pain or muscle weakness
  - Aspiration and the inability to handle secretions (The cuffed tube allows the trachea to be sealed off from the esophagus and its refluxing contents).

Advantages of Tracheostomy over Translaryngeal Intubation

- Reduces patient discomfort
- Reduces need for sedation
- Improves ability to maintain orodental and bronchial hygiene
- Improves patient appearance and overall safety
- Eliminates the ongoing risks of sinusitis and oral, nasal, and pharyngeal injuries[9]
- Reduces risk of glottic trauma
- Reduces dead space and work of breathing (WOB)[10]
- Reduces the risk of ventilator-associated pneumonia[11,12]
- Facilitates oral communication and speech
- Augments process of weaning from ventilatory support
- Lower incidence of tube obstruction
- Easy changes of cannula and better airway protection
- Better preserved swallowing, which allows earlier oral feeding[13-15]
- Improves patient mobility
- Eases disposition of long-term care facility/ home care.

Advantages of Percutaneous Tracheostomy

- Minimally invasive procedure and usually performed at the bedside in ICU therefore the risks of shifting the patient to operation room are avoided
- Has significant cost benefits compared to open procedure
- May be associated with a reduced risk of bleeding and infection
- Success rates of more than 98% have been reported
- Mortality related to the procedure is less than 0.5%
- Complications are less to those following open procedure and occur in 5-15% of patients

- Bronchoscopic guidance may further reduce the complication rate
- Incidence of tracheal stenosis are less than open methods
- Stoma scar is quite small (button scar) and is esthetically more favorable (Fig. 3.2).

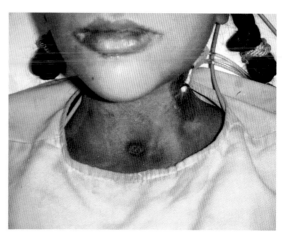

Fig. 3.2: Percutaneous tracheostomy scar (Button scar) after 24 hours of decannulation

Timing of Tracheostomy

Though there are no definite guidelines indicating the exact time interval for the formation of tracheostomy after endotracheal intubation, however, the timing of tracheostomy has changed over recent years and is influenced by the indications for the procedure. Two decades back tracheostomy was considered 'early' if it was performed before three weeks of translaryngeal intubation. Previous recommendations to avoid tracheostomy for as long as 14-21 days are now obsolete.[16] Only one report, in which the authors noted methodological limitations, did not support the use of early tracheostomy.[17] In the otorhinolaryngology literature, however, the performance of tracheostomy to protect the larynx from intubation damage has been recommended within 3 days of intubation.[9] This recommendation is based on the fact that the visually observed mucosal damage to the larynx and cords is maximal in 3-7 days and if tube is removed within this period complete healing of injuries occur.[18] If translaryngeal intubation is continued for longer than one week, the visually assessed damage progresses with scar formation and functional abnormality in voice occur with increasing frequency.[19] Rumbak and colleagues[20] defined early tracheostomy as placement of PDT by day-2. In their study, 60 patients underwent tracheostomy in each group. There was a significant difference between the early tracheostomy groups and prolonged translaryngeal intubation group in outcome measures and yielded important evidence suggesting that early tracheostomy should be considered in any patient who is unlikely to wean early. Their study was strengthened by the standard weaning and sedation practices. The authors reported remarkable findings in support of early tracheostomy, safety of PDT, and lack of complications when the procedure is performed by qualified clinicians.

In a recent survey of 152 French ICUs, Blot et al found that in two thirds of ICUs the tracheostomy was performed after a mean period of 7 days of translaryngeal intubation.[21] The likelihood of significant laryngeal injury with the continued use of translaryngeal intubation for prolonged period versus frequency of tracheal stoma or tracheostomy related complications must be weighed. More recently, in a systemic review and meta-analysis, Griffith and colleagues concluded that early tracheostomy significantly reduce duration of artificial ventilation and length of stay in ICU.[22] However, the timing of tracheostomy had no effect on mortality or on development of pneumonia. In a randomized and controlled clinical study, Kollef and coworkers compared early (less than 48 hours) versus late (after 14 days) tracheostomy in patients with respiratory failure.[23] Significant reduction in mortality, pneumonia and duration of mechanical ventilation was observed in the group who had early tracheostomy. However, these results have not been confirmed in subsequent clinical trials. Early tracheostomy at seven days of translaryngeal intubation is thought to be appropriate for patients in whom weaning from ventilation and extubation are not likely before two weeks.

The decision to place a tracheostomy should be individualized, balancing the patient's wishes, expected recovery course, risk of continued translaryngeal intubation and the potential risk of tracheostomy. The individualization of tracheostomy timing has been termed the "anticipatory approach".[24-27] If a translaryngeally intubated patient remains ventilator dependent for a week, a tracheostomy can be considered and the decision to perform the procedure would depend on (i) the patient's likelihood of benefiting from tracheostomy and (ii) anticipated duration of continued ventilatory support.[28] Patients with progressive and irreversible causes of respiratory failure, such as amytrophic lateral sclerosis or cervical spine injuries, do not benefit from a trial of weaning, so a tracheostomy can be placed as soon as stabilization occurs after endotracheal intubation. The anticipatory approach depends on the ability of clinicians to predict the duration of mechanical ventilation.

CONCLUSION

The introduction of bedside percutaneous tracheostomy techniques and their reported benefits over open tracheostomy have led to formation of elective tracheostomy earlier in the course of critical illness. The patients who may require prolonged ventilatory support for respiratory failure and can not be weaned within 7-10 days are the suitable candidates for tracheostomy. Patients with severe trauma or intracranial bleeds who are unconscious and not likely to awaken within a week may benefit with early tracheostomy.[29,30]

REFERENCES

1. Heffner JE, Hess D. Tracheostomy management in the chronically ventilated patient. Clin Chest Med 2001;22:55-69.

2. Stauffer JL, Olson DE, Petty TL. Complications and consequences of endotracheal intubation and tracheostomy. A prospective study of 150 critically ill adult patients. Am J Med 1981;70:65-76.

3. Plummer AL, Gracey DR. Consensus conference on artificial airways inpatients receiving mechanical ventilation. Chest 1989;96:178-80.

4. Friedman Y. Indications, timing, techniques, and complications of tracheostomy in the critically ill patient. Curr Opin Crit Care 1996;2:47-53.

5. Gründling M, Quintel M. Percutaneous dilational tracheostomy. Indications—techniques—complications. Anaesthesist 2005;54:929-41.

6. Sousa A, Nunes T, Roque Farinha R, Bandeira T. Tracheostomy: Indications and complications in paediatric patients. Rev Port Pneumol. 2009;15:227-39.

7. Zenk J, Fyrmpas G, Zimmermann T, Koch M, Constantinidis J, Iro H. Tracheostomy in young patients: Indications and long-term outcome. Eur Arch Otorhinolaryngol 2009;266:705-11.

8. Groves DS, Durbin CG Jr. Tracheostomy in the critically ill: Indications, timing and techniques. Curr Opin Crit Care 2007;13:90-7.

9. Durbin CG. Indications for and timing of tracheostomy. Respir Care 2005;50:483-7.

10. Jaeger JM, Littlewood KA, Durbin CG Jr. The role of tracheostomy in weaning from mechanical ventilation. Respir Care 2002;47:469-80.

11. Kollef MH. The prevention of ventilator-associated pneumonia. N Eng J Med 1999;340:627-34.

12. Kollof MH, Ahrens TS, Shannon W. Clinical predictors and outcomes for patients requiring tracheostomy in the intensive care unit. Crit Care Med 1999;27:1714-20.

13. Elpern EH, Scott MG, Petro L, Ries MH. Pulmonary aspiration in mechanically ventilated patients with tracheostomies. Chest 1994;105:563-6.

14. Devita MA, Spierer-Rundback MS. Swallowing disorders in patients with prolonged intubations or tracheostomy tubes. Crit Care Med 1990;18:1328-32.

15. Tolep K, Getch CL, Criner GJ. Swallowing dysfunction in patients receiving prolonged mechanical ventilation. Chest 1996;109:167-72.

16. Marsh HM, Gillespie DJ, Baumgartner AE. Timing of tracheostomy in the critically ill patient. Chest 1989;96:190-3.

17. Sugarman HJ, Wolfe L, Pasquale MD, Rogers FB, O'Malley KF, et al. Multicenter randomized, prospective trial of early tracheostomy. J Trauma 1997;43:741-7.

18. Colice GL. Resolution of laryngeal injury following translaryngeal intubation. Am Rev Respir Dis 1992;145:361-4.

19. Whited RE. A prospective study of laryngotracheal sequelae in long-term intubation. Laryngoscope 1984;94:367-77.

20. Rumbak MJ, Newton M, Truncale T, Schwartz SW, Adams JW, Hazard PB. A prospective, randomized study comparing early percutaneous dilational tracheotomy to prolonged translaryngeal intubation (delayed tracheotomy) in critically ill medical patients. Crit Care Med 2004,32:1689-94.

21. Blot F, Melot C. Indications, timing, and techniques of tracheostomy in 152 French ICUs. Chest 2005;127:1347-52.

22. Griffiths J, Barber VS, Morgan L, Young JD. Systemic review and meta-analysis of studies and the timing of tracheostomy in adult patients undergoing artificial ventilation. Br Med J 2005;330:1243-7.

23. Kollef MH, Ahrens TS, Shannon W. Clinical predictors and outcomes for patients requiring tracheostomy in the intensive care unit. Cri Care Med 1999;27:1714-20

24. Heffner JE. Timing of tracheostomy in mechanically ventilated patients. Am Rev Respir Dis 1993;147:768-71.

25. Plummer AL, Gracey DR. Consensus conference on artificial airways in patients receiving mechanical ventilation. Chest 1989;96:178-84.

26. Heffner JE. Medical indications for tracheostomy. Chest 1989;96:186-90.

27. Heffner JE. Timing of tracheostomy in ventilator dependent patients. Clin Chest Med 1991;12:611-25.

28. Heffner JE. Tracheostomy application and timing. Clin Chest Med 2003;24:389-98.

29. Kapadia FN, Bajan KB, Raje KV. Airway accidents in intubated intensive care unit patients: An epidemiological study. Crit Care Med 2000;28:659-64.

30. Major KM, Hui T, Wilson MT, Gaon MD, Shabot MM, Marguilies DR. Objective indications for early tracheostomy after blunt head trauma. Am J Surg 2003;186:615-9.

Standard Surgical Tracheostomy

Isha Tyagi, Sushil P Ambesh

Though percutaneous dilatational tracheostomy (PDT) has become a standard technique in critical care medicine, surgical tracheostomy may be asked for difficult patients like with thick and short neck or deformed cervical anatomy, laryngeal tumors etc. Overall, the indications for tracheostomy (described elsewhere) remain the same as they used to be whether it be percutaneous technique or surgical.

Tracheotomy though a very simple procedure and at times life saving as we know but there are few small tips which any new surgeon must learn before attempting to perform tracheostomy. We strongly recommend no surgeon should perform tracheostomy himself without a prior experience of assisting except in few emergency situations where it is life saving.

Here is a description of the surgical procedure which may be quite useful for surgeons who have no prior exposure to this procedure and experienced surgeon may still find some useful tips. A detailed description of relevant anatomy of larynx and the trachea is given in Chapter 2.

INSTRUMENTS FOR TRACHEOTOMY

Several instruments that are required during surgical tracheostomy are shown in Table 4.1. For optimal

Table 4.1: Equipments for surgical tracheostomy
• Knife – '15' size blade for the skin incision and '11' or '12' size blade for the tracheotomy.
• Alley's forceps – 2
• Artery forceps – 4
• Lengenbeck's retractor – 2
• Cricoid/tracheal hook – 1
• Trousseau's tracheal dilator – 1
• Tracheostomy tube (High volume low pressure cuff) – 2
• Electrocautery
• Sterile suction catheter
• Sterile aqueous lubricating jelly
• Sterile adaptor
• Twill tape
• Head light

visualization of the surgical field good lighting and suction are essential.

The cricoid or tracheal hook is particularly important in patients who have short stature with a thick neck in whom the trachea may lie deep into the soft tissues and may even reside behind the sternum. The tracheal hook will allow the surgeon to bring the trachea more into the operative field. A syringe is used to check the integrity of the cuff and pilot balloon of tracheostomy tube. The tracheal dilator is essential for enlarging the tracheal incision to accommodate the tracheostomy tube. Application of the sterile jelly over the tracheostomy tube facilitates its insertion through the newly formed tracheal stoma.

PATIENT POSITIONING

Elective tracheostomy is usually performed in the operating theater on a patient under general anesthesia. However, bedside tracheostomy can be performed by the experienced surgeons in the intensive care unit. Usually the airway is secured with cuffed endotracheal tube; however, in patients with upper airway obstructive lesions surgical tracheostomy may be performed under local anesthesia and light (or no) sedation. Though practice of administering prophylactic antibiotics varies from hospital to hospital however, at our center we prefer intravenous injection of Augmentin 1.2 gm (Amoxycillin 1gm + Clauvulanic acid 250 mg) about 30 min prior to skin incision.

A written informed consent must be obtained from the patient (if possible) or next of kin. The positioning of the patient is crucial for surgical tracheostomy. The patient is placed supine on the operating table with the neck moderately extended by placing a pillow or rolled sheet transversely under the shoulders. One must ensure that occiput is resting on the head ring firmly. Hyperextension of neck may cause neck injuries and is contraindicated in patients with proven or suspected cervical spine injury. One should be careful especially in individuals with thick and short neck. Extension of the neck will bring in a certain length of trachea from thorax into neck thereby providing more operating space to the surgeon. Extension of neck will also bring trachea closure to skin and thereby decreasing the depth for dissection. It is a good practice to keep the extension of the neck to the last part of the preparation in nonintubated patient as the hyperextension of neck is very uncomfortable for a conscious patient to maintain it for a long time; and especially if there is some degree of upper airway obstruction. In these situations patient's cooperation is essential. Situation can be eased by positioning of such patients to hyperextension near the end of the procedure. If possible, the operating table should be placed at approximately 15° of reverse Trendenlenburg position to decrease venous bleeding in the surgical field. However, it should be noted that in this position the patient is more prone to air embolism if a major venous injury occurs and patient is not receiving positive pressure ventilation.

PART PREPARATION AND DRAPING

Part preparation is done just like in any other surgical procedure. With the patient positioned prior to being prepped, the surgeon should carefully review the superficial landmarks of the regional anatomy, including the tip of the chin, thyroid cartilage, cricoid cartilage and the suprasternal notch. Draping of the part is done using four towels one on each side of the neck. In case patient is intubated then endotracheal (ET) tube should be taken over the head so that surgeon gets a clear field and anesthesiologist has ease of withdrawing it whenever required. In case sticky drape is used it has to be ensured that it is not sticking to the ET tube otherwise it will hamper with the withdrawing of the ET tube.

The marked incision site is now infiltrated with 2% lignocaine with 1:200,000 adrenaline solution. Be careful not to exceed the dose of lignocaine (7 mg/kg) and not to inject directly into the vessel. Sufficient time should be given for the adrenaline to have its effect. Infiltration also helps in providing pain relief in the postoperative period. It is always better to inject a few drops of 4% lignocaine into the trachea before giving incision on trachea. This will reduce the cough reflex while the tracheostomy tube is inserted and it also reconfirms the position of trachea by throwing air bubbles into syringe if slight negative pressure is created in the syringe.

It is a good idea to check the tracheostomy tube. Air is injected into the tracheal cuff to ensure there are no leaks. All the air is then removed from the tracheal cuff and pilot balloon; and blunt tipped obturator is inserted into the tracheostomy tube. Water soluble lubricating jelly is applied on the cuff. The size of the tube selected depends on the size of the airway. It is always better to have one size smaller tube at the standby. Generally, tracheostomy tube should occupy approximately three-fourths of the tracheal lumen. There is no correlation between airway size and the patient's age, height or weight. However, women have a smaller larynx and smaller trachea than men.

OPERATIVE TECHNIQUE

Marking the incision is very important in tracheotomy for the ease of procedure. First mark the key landmarks. Prominence of cricoid cartilage and sternal notch is palpated and marked first. Mid point of these two marks is the right place for making incision. It is marked by drawing a horizontal line preferably by a marking pen or betadine at this level. The skin is incised transversely with the knife. Length of incision varies according to the experience of the surgeon. It is better for a beginner to give incision of about 5-6 cm in length (Fig. 4.1A). As the surgeon becomes experienced he can change to smaller incisions according to his experience. Ideally incision should be large enough to allow dissection with ease, particularly in individuals with short and thick neck.[1,2]

Incision is deepened and platysma is incised in the same line and the incision is carried down to the deep fascia which is also incised in the same line (Fig. 4.1B). At this stage anterior jugular veins are encountered and they can be ligated, coagulated or retraced laterally according to the situation. One must be meticulous about hemostasis in this area. The fascia between the strap muscles (sternohyoid, omohyoid and sternohyoid) is divided vertically with scissors or electrocautery. The midline is identified and two side muscles are separated by dissection. It is very important that we remain in the midline

as the dissection plane in the midline is relatively avascular and safe.

At this point a new surgeon must realize that trachea is deeper than we expect so he must divide all the tissue layers in the same line of incision to get maximum advantage of the large incision. The dissected muscles are retracted laterally thereby exposing the trachea which is covered by pretracheal fascia .It is usually possible to retract thyroid isthmus superiorly but ideally it is recommended to divide it in the midline by applying clamps from the superior side. The cut ends are ligated using a 2-0 absorbable suture material. It is then retracted laterally along with the neck muscles. Retraction of thyroid gland is usually difficult as it is attached to the pretracheal fascia and it will have to be separated from the pretracheal fascia to be able to retract which will again lead to bleeding. The authors, therefore, always prefer to ligate it rather than retract. In individuals with thick neck division of the isthmus is all the more recommended. Then there is one more situation which surgeon must keep in mind about the inferior thyroid veins which may come in the operation field and at times can create problems. It is best to coagulate them by a bipolar even before they bleed.

Division of the isthmus is important to define better surgical anatomy of trachea and to ensure formation of tracheal stoma between second and third tracheal rings. Higher placement of tracheostomy may result in subglottic tracheal stenosis while lower placement may cause erosion of the innominate artery. Division of the isthmus also allows us to estimate the tracheal diameter in order to select appropriate size of tracheostomy tube. Clamps are placed on either side of the intended area of division and the isthmus is sequentially clamped, divided and ligated in three or four steps.

Cricoid hook is very useful to pull the trachea in to the operating field if visibility of the site of tracheotomy is not proper. It was a tradition to make a tracheal wall flap and stitch this flap to the

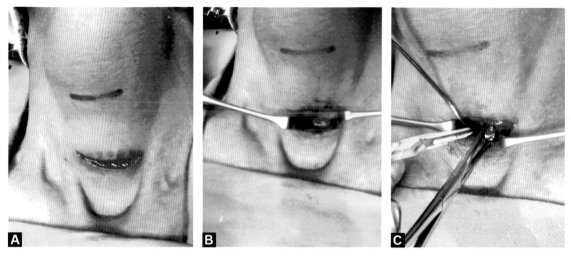

Figs 4.1A to C: (A) Skin incision **(B)** Platysma divided **(C)** Tracheal flap excised

skin (Fig. 4.1C). It had the advantage of allowing easy change of tube but it had many problems as at times the suture would cut through the trachea and the flap would fall back making the tracheostomy tube insertion even more difficult. Besides this it has also been associated with increased incidence of long term tracheal stenosis. It is, therefore, no longer practiced. The ideal incision for tracheotomy should be neatly given in a circular fashion. We first make a U-shaped incision based superiorly, hold the free edge of the cartilage with an Alley's forceps and then joining the two limbs of U. This way we are able to remove the cut piece of the tracheal cartilage safely and chances of it getting sucked into the trachea are minimized.

INSERTION OF TRACHEOSTOMY TUBE

If the patient is intubated anesthesiologist is asked to deflate the ET tube cuff and slowly withdraw the ET tube under direct vision to free the tracheal stoma site. When the tip of the ET tube is just barely visible in the cephalad portion of the tracheal incision and tracheal lumen comes in view, tracheal stoma is opened by introducing the Trousseau dilator (Fig. 4.2A). An appropriate size tracheostomy tube is now quickly introduced and its obturator is

removed (Fig. 4.2B). Following placement of the tracheostomy tube aspirate the tracheal secretions by introducing a suction catheter through tracheostomy tube. Aspiration of the tracheal secretions assures that the tracheostomy tube has been placed correctly in the tracheal airway. The tracheal cuff is then inflated with a minimal occluding volume. If the patient was under anesthesia then anesthesiologist is asked to shift the gas circuit to the tracheostomy while surgeon maintains it firmly in position. Correct placement of tracheostomy must also be verified by monitoring the end-tidal carbon dioxide and airway pressure. Cuff prevents any aspiration of secretions once the ET tube is withdrawn. Cuff pressure is very important if one has to prevent any tracheal damage.[3] In intensive care units where patient remains tracheostomized for a long time cuff pressure is all the more important. The blood supply of the tracheal mucosa is vulnerable to excessive cuff pressure and studies have shown that inflation pressure exceeding 30 cm H_2O (22 mm Hg) will produce ischemia.[4] There are many devices available today which can measure the cuff pressure and they should be used while inflating the cuff. A high pressure even in a low pressure

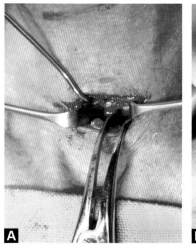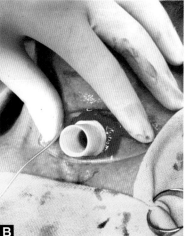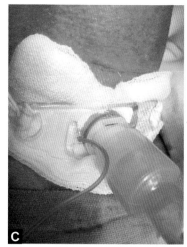

Figs 4.2A to C: (A) Trousseau dilator **(B)** Tracheostomy tube inserted **(C)** Tracheostomy dressed

cuff can impair capillary blood flow in the mucosa and can therefore lead to mucosal damage.

The lateral edges of the tracheostomy can be sutured to skin edges as this facilitates tube change. It is usually done in children where replacing the tube is difficult. In adults, however, it is difficult to put these sutures as the cartilage may be calcified and sutures have a tendency to cut through. It is better to use monofilament nylon in adults and Vicryl in children for this purpose.

With the tracheostomy tube in satisfactory position, the tracheal incision is very loosely closed around the tracheostomy tube and it is better to close only the skin with 2-3 monofilament sutures. A tight closure can result in subcutaneous emphysema as some amount of air always leaks around the tracheostomy tube, therefore, it should be allowed to pass out. A cotton "twill tape" is used to secure the tracheostomy tube around the neck.

Patient neck is then brought into neutral position by removing the shoulder support bags. It is mandatory to do this before tying the tape around neck other wise the tapes will become loose and tube will have a tendency to fall out. A soft pad is cut halfway and inserted under the tube to prevent the flanges of the tracheostomy tube coming in contact with the skin (Fig. 4.2C). Dressing should not be packed into the wound as this would result in trapping the air in soft tissues and will cause wound breakdown and postoperative scarring.

Changing of Tracheostomy Tube

The surgically formed tracheostomy track takes about 72 hours to form, therefore, change of tube should be avoided during this period. However, it may sometimes become necessary to change it before this period. At times the tube may get displaced into soft tissue or it may get blocked. A good nursing care of tracheotomized patient is therefore very important in the immediate post operative period to avoid these problems. It is better to have a tracheostomy set ready if there is a need to change the tracheostomy tube before the said time. It is a golden tip to put a suction catheter or a hollow bougie through the tracheostomy tube *in situ* and use it as a guide to introduce the new tube.

COMPLICATIONS

Surgical tracheostomy is very basic but at times life threatening complications can occur during or soon after the surgery. Late complications should not occur in present day practice however, some times tracheal stenosis or tracheomalacia can occur.[5-7]

Intra-operative Complications

• Intra-operative Hemorrhage
• Airway fire
• Injury to trachea and larynx
• Injury to paratracheal structures
• Air embolism
• Apnea
• Cardiac arrest

Early Postoperative

• Early postoperative subcutaneous emphysema
• Pneumothorax/pneumomediastinum
• Tube displacement
• Tube blockage (crusts)
• Wound infection

Late

• Tracheal necrosis
• Secondary hemorrhage
• Swallowing problems
• Late postoperative hemorrhage
• Granuloma formation
• Tracheoesophageal fistula
• Difficult decannulation
• Tracheocutaneous fistula
• Laryngotracheal stenosis
• Tracheostomy scar

Preoperative complications are primarily surgical problems. The early postoperative problems largely depend on the proper nursing care. A good nursing care will prevent most of these problems. Late complications are due to preoperative injuries to the air way which were not detected at the time of surgery or were overlooked and again poor post operative nursing care can also lead to some of the late problems. Late complications will not be described here.

Coagulation disorders should be kept in mind especially while performing tracheostomy on a critically ill patient and it must be corrected as far as possible preoperatively. Preoperative bleeding can be reduced if surgery is being done under local anesthesia by allowing sufficient time after the injection for the adrenaline to have its effect. Another common source for the significant bleeding is the thyroid isthmus and the anterior jugular veins. Injury to large vessels can be avoided by dissecting in the midline and not going lateral to the trachea. The anterior jugular veins if they come in the operating field should be meticulously ligated and cut. The veins even when injured during surgery often do not bleed immediately as they remain compressed by the force of retraction and may bleed later even after few hours of surgery.

REFERENCES

1. Bernard AC, Kenady DE. Conventional surgical tracheostomy as the preferred method of airway management. J Oral Maxillofac Surg 1999;57:310-15.
2. Claudia R, Bassel M. Tracheostomy Practitioner: Tracheostomy a multiprofessional handbook. Cambridge University Press, Greenwich Medical Media Limited 2004.
3. Camargo MF, Andrade AP, Cardoso FP, Melo MH. Analysis of the intracuff pressures of intensive care patients. Rev Assoc Med Bras 2006;52:405-8.
4. Seegobin RD, Van Hasselt GL. Endotracheal cuff pressure and tracheal mucosa blood flow: Endoscopic studies of effects of four large volume cuffs. Br Med J 1984; 228:965-8.
5. Amusa YB, Akinpelu VO, Fadiora SO, Agbakwuru EA. Tracheostomy in surgical practice: Experience in a Nigerian tertiary hospital. West Afr J Med 2004;23:32-4.
6. Lewis RJ. Tracheostomies. Indications, timing, and complications. Clin Chest Med. 1992;13(1):137-49.
7. Walts PA, Murthy SC, DeCamp MM. Techniques of surgical tracheostomy. Clin Chest Med 2003;24:413-22.

Cricothyroidotomy

Giulio Frova, Massimiliano Sorbello

INTRODUCTION

Cricothyroidotomy or more simply, cricothyrotomy, is an invasive procedure also defined as thyrocricotomy, intercricothyrotomy, inferior laryngotomy, coniotomy and minitracheostomy; it represents the best way to perform a direct airway access at the level of cricothyroid membrane, both as elective or emergency procedure. Accordingly to the inserted cannula diameter, some Authors [1] distinguish a true cricothyrotomy from the simple cricothyroid membrane puncture; on the practical point of view, indeed, and in this chapter, both maneuvers will be considered as equivalent aspects of cricothyrotomy, being equal in terms of aims, though different in terms of efficacy.

Cricothyrotomy is a well and long time known procedure, yet described many centuries ago and re-valuated by Brantigan's and Grow's papers[2,3] demonstrating how wrong was the concept that a subglottic stenosis had to be considered a natural consequence of the subcricothyroideal space opening.

A pivotal role for cricothyrotomy diffusion in the last 15 years was also played by international difficult airway guidelines, unanimously considering this maneuver as a life-saving procedure in case of precipitating hypoxia after all possible attempts to grant ventilation and oxygenation with non-invasive techniques.[4]

Cricothyrotomy represents the only invasive procedures suggested for the adult patient by the American Society of Anesthesiologists (ASA),[5] Italian Society of Anesthesia, Resuscitation, and Intensive Therapy (SIAARTI),[6] International Liaison Committee on Resuscitation (ILCOR),[7] and **European Resuscitation Council** (ERC)[8] algorithms after repeated intubation attempts failure and in case of impossible ventilation/oxygenation of the patient (Can't Ventilate – Can't Intubate scenario) in operation theater, in intensive care unit, in emergency department and in the out-of-hospital setting. Emergency tracheostomy being less and less indicated today.

Indications

The main indication for cricothyrotomy is represented by severe hypoxic emergency, aimed to obtain oxygenation whenever both intubation attempts fail and use of extraglottic devices is no more effective or impossible. Conversely, elective indications for cricothyrotomy are:

a. Ventilation in case of maxillo-facial severe trauma or burns preventing laryngoscopy performance or use of facial and laryngeal mask.

b. Patients in which intubation is not possible because of:
   - Glottic edema
   - Pharyngeal or tracheobronchial hemorrhage
   - Severe cervical trauma or cervical instable fracture
   - Skull base fractures
   - Airway obstruction by foreign bodies
   - Trismus
c. Postoperatory tracheobronchial toilette.
d. Asphyxia prophylaxis in case of laryngeal obstruction, when anesthesia and surgery are scheduled.[9]

A paper by Erlandson and coworkers[10] studying cricothyrotomy indications in 77 cases reported: (a) facial or neck trauma 26%, (b) tracheobronchial hemorrhage 4%, (c) failed intubation (hemorrhage 19%, cervical trauma 19%, trismus 8%, other causes 14%), (d) after tracheal puncture for CV–CI 9%. Fortune and Coworkers[11] reported the performance of extra-hospital cricothyroidotomy in 56 trauma patients; the primary indications were facial fractures with deformities (32%), blood or gastric contents in the airway (30%), traumatic obstruction (7%) and can not ventilate can not intubate (CV-CI) situations (11%).

The only absolute contraindication for cricothyrotomy is represented by the possibility of other non-invasive procedures; relative contraindications might be considered children less than 5 years old (in which the simple tracheal puncture or surgical tracheotomy are indicated), laryngeal tumors or trauma, acute laryngeal pathology or anatomical barriers such as hematoma, emphysema or goiter.

Incidence

Cricothyrotomy and in a broad sense the rapid tracheal access incidence is almost unknown, with variable data ranging from very low values in operation theater up to almost higher values in the out-of-hospital setting.

Indeed incidence trends depend not only on the context in which cricothyrotomy might be performed, but also on the role (physicians or paramedics) of operators;[12,13] furtherly, the growing diffusion of extraglottic devices could actually limit out-of-hospital cricothyrotomy requirements,[14] despite the increasing number of commercially available kits.

According to the authors' personal experience, the dramatic clinical scenario leading to cricothyrotomy seems to occur very rarely in operating theater (about 5 pts per million of anesthetics or 0.0005%). This value is lower than the classically reported rate of 0.01% (that is 100 patients per million of anesthetics);[15] on the other hand, it remains quite clear that cricothyrotomy occurs at least one thousand times more frequently (0.5%, that is 5000 cricothyrotomies per million of patients) in emergency wards[16] and even more (up to 14%) in out-of-hospital setting, whenever respiratory emergency management is performed by paramedics and non-physicians.[17] Retrospective studies suggest, in fact, that cricothyrotomy occurs in about 1% of all emergency airways.[18]

A pivotal role for cricothyrotomy incidence reduction in elective or emergency setting was surely played by difficult airway management guidelines diffusion; the use of Laryngeal Mask Airway as a successful bridge to secure the airway in alternative to facial mask in impossible ventilation situations might have contributed to the reduction of both critical accidents and cricothyrotomy rate as life-rescuing procedure.[4,17,19,20]

ANATOMY

Cricothyroideal membrane extends from the lower edge of thyroid cartilage down to the upper edge of the cricoid cartilage; it is shaped as an enlarged trapezoid, poorly vascular and corresponding to the only complete ring of laryngotracheal structure that increases the posterior wall protection.[21] It remains superficial (0.5-1 cm depth), being covered by sole skin, subcutaneous tissue and a thin fascia.

With respect to its dimensions (8 -10 mm height, 22-30 mm width), the risk-free surface useful for puncture has a lower extension, equivalent to the lower half of the membrane and a few millimeters laterally to the midline. The superior third is in fact considered at risk, because both vocal cords are located 1 cm above the membrane and because of transversal cricothyroideal arteries, thin branches of superior thyroideal arteries running vertically in the lateral area of the membrane in more than 50% of normal subjects. Thyroid gland is usually located below the membrane, but in 40% of population the pyramidal lobe might interest the left side of the membrane itself; for all these reasons it is suggested to use cannulas not larger than 8 mm outer diameter.

In normal subjects the cricothyroid membrane is easily located by simple palpation: using the fore finger to explore the anterior neck region below the chin region by identification of hyoid bone and of thyroideal prominence (*Adam's apple*), below which the membrane is perceived as a depression, before rising up again on the cricoid cartilage.

Usually the cricothyroid membrane is located 1.5-2 transversal fingers below thyroideal prominence: when grabbing thyroid cartilage between the thumb and the third finger, the fore finger's tip deepens caudally into the membrane's location; if stretching the skin with the two fingers in the same position, a kind of groove appears in the membrane's location.

Procedure and Techniques

Three techniques have been identified to perform rapid airway access:
a. Needle (catheter over the needle) puncture
   - Low pressure ventilation
   - Transtracheal jet ventilation (TTJV)
b. Surgical (or *opened*) cricothyrotomy

c. Percutaneous cricothyrotomy
   - According to Seldinger's technique
   - Other techniques

Cricothyroideal membrane puncture is the easiest way to perform a rapid airway access, and difficult airways management guidelines do not strictly suggest the best way (either tracheal puncture or cricothyrotomy) to perform this life saving procedure in the CV – CI patient.

The simple cricothyroideal membrane puncture is widespread because of the easy availability of large bore catheters over the needle (13-14 G, that is about 1.5 mm inner diameter), either simple vascular access catheters (which might kink and slip out, causing airway loss) or dedicated reinforced and bent catheters. In United Kingdom this maneuver is yet officially taught to ambulance paramedics to be used with low pressure oxygenation,[22] despite strong evidence [14] indicates this technique to be poorly effective in delivering a 2 l min^{-1} via a 13 G catheter, if not unuseful or even potentially harmful, because the small diameter prevents expiration.[13]

Several cricothyroideal membrane puncture dedicated catheter over the needle kits are commercially available: *Ravussin*® catheter[23] in the different versions 1.3 mm ID (2.0 mm OD) and 1.7 mm ID (2.3 mm OD); *ETAC* reinforced catheter (*Emergency Transtracheal Airway Catheter*® – Cook) in the different versions 2.0 mm ID (2.7 mm OD); *Patil Emergency Cricothyrotomy Catheter*® (Cook) in the different versions 2.0 mm ID (3.3 mm OD) and 3.0 mm ID (4.2 mm OD); both of them are dedicated reinforced catheters so to avoid kinking after entering the airway.

Ventilation through such a small diameter catheters with low pressure ventilation allows oxygenation only, not ventilation, and prevents adequate expiration; on the other hand, after emergency setting, a Seldinger guide wire passed through the existing cannula might allow a larger bore cannula insertion. Between catheter-over-needle devices, the *Quicktrach Teleflex®* (larger cannulas mounted over large bore needles) represents alternative choices discussed below.

Whatever the catheter-over-needle system, all should be inserted through the membrane with a 30° angle with respect to the skin[1] and inserted until clear airway identification by free air aspiration in a liquid prefilled syringe.

Any catheter-over-needle approach, indeed, represents a low efficacy system to provide ventilation, furtherly being affected by another important limitation that is connection with manual self-expandable balloon or low pressure breathing circuit which might be often difficult and time consuming.[24]

The following are considered as possible connections (Fig. 5.1):
1. 2.5 ml syringe to be connected distally to the catheter and proximally with a standard 15 mm endotracheal tube connector after piston removal.
2. Straight connection between catheter and pediatric tracheal tube standard 15 mm connector.
3. 10 ml syringe to be connected distally to the catheter and proximally with an inserted cuffed tracheal tube after piston removal and cuff inflation.

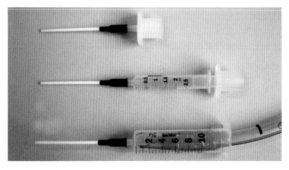

Fig. 5.1: Suggested connections between needle and apparatus

The only way to grant effective ventilation through a catheter over the needle is represented by a high pressure apparatus connected via LuerLock, as stated by Benumof.[25] Now a days simple devices are commercially available, providing a driving pressure control which could be maintained at about 20 psi.[1] Risks deriving from these instruments are represented by high inflation overpressures, which might cause lung hyper-expansion, pneumothorax and dangerous false airway routes, especially in presence of hindered expiration. A cyclic disconnection or a stopcock to be temporarily opened, are suggested to allow airway pressure release.

Surgical (open) Cricothyrotomy

Though more difficult than original definition of "restaurant tracheostomy" (It can be performed in a restaurant with a jack knife and the barrel of a pen for a tube)[2] this quite simple technique allows the direct placement of a small size cuffed tracheal tube through an incision in the cricothyroideal membrane. The surgical approach can establish an airway in less than 40 sec.[26] The potential risk of hemorrhage and laryngeal trauma seems greater with this technique if compared with other, but, similarly to surgical vs percutaneous tracheostomy debate, the relatively high incidence of many problems (such as tube misplacement, bleeding, necessity of blood vessels ligature) described in previous papers[27] seems to be lower in recent studies.[28] Complications rate with percutaneous procedure vs surgical technique seems identical.[29]

The only advantages of this technique are represented by quicker time to perform the procedure and by the airway protection in terms of aspiration risks thanking to the use of a cuffed tube instead of uncuffed cannulas largely used in the percutaneous procedure.

The knowledge of the surgical procedure might be a duty and an advantage for every anesthesiologist and emergency physician, even because the necessary equipment is very simple, ranging from a scalpel only[13] to the more complex equipment described by Helm.[30] In our experience, the necessary equipment to perform a safe surgical cricothyrotomy might be limited to a scalpel, a curved-tip forceps (Klemmer), an intubating metal semi-rigid stylet and a cuffed 5.0-6.0 ID endotracheal tube (Fig. 5.2), avoiding the need of any dedicated set in the operating theater. Conversely, a dedicated surgical kit should be available in the out-of-operation theatre setting, even if, for practical reasons, it is often substituted by available commercial kits for percutaneous cricothyrotomy.

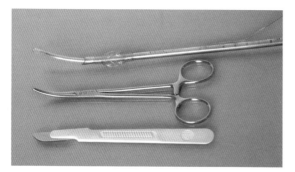

Fig. 5.2: Components of surgical set: Scalpel, curved forceps, stylet and small size cuffed tube

The procedure should be performed with head in hyperextension, as Gerling and coworkers [31] demonstrated that the risk of worsening a cervical spine lesion is insignificant. Operator's position is indifferent, both on right or left side, and at the head side of the patient.

What remains mandatory is patient's larynx fixation: this can be obtained by fixing thyroid cartilage with thumb and third finger (Fig. 5.3) of the non-dominating hand (usually left hand if standing at the right or at the head of the patient), while identifying the cricothyroideal membrane with the fore finger, leaving the dominating hand free to perform the procedure. The same efficacy, in the authors' experience, has been provided by a

left side standing position, with combined left hand thumb and third finger immobilization of cricoid cartilage and first tracheal rings and procedure performance by right hand (Fig. 5.4).

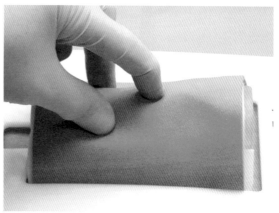

Fig. 5.3: Immobilization of the thyroid during procedure

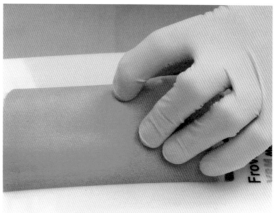

Fig. 5.4: Immobilization of the cricoid during procedure

A midline, less than 2 cm vertical or horizontal[13] incision is performed, followed by careful smooth dissection using the forceps down to reach the membrane, which can be transversally cut or, more simply, perforated by the same forceps, closed and gripped close to the tip (Fig. 5.5). The forceps arms are then gently opened in a vertical direction and again in a transversal direction, followed by

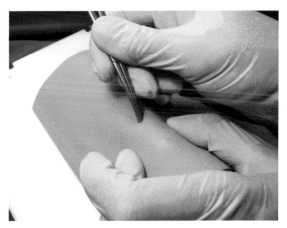

Fig. 5.5: Use of a curved forceps

intubation stylet (the tip moderately downwards bent) insertion. The stylet should proceed smoothly and obstacle-free into the trachea before railroading the previously lubricated endotracheal cuffed tube over it. The tube's correct position is then checked, the cuff inflated and oxygenation might be started. A 5-6 mm ID cuffed endotracheal tube offers many advantages: no high pressure sources are needed, exhalation is generally effective with very low risks of lung injury and up to 15 l min^{-1} ventilation rates (instead of 4-6 l min^{-1} with a 4-6 mm ID *uncuffed* tube) can be easily obtained [32], allowing not only oxygenation but also ventilation.

No more than 1-3 minutes are usually required to perform the maneuver,[12] accordingly to operator's experience, with a range between more than two minutes in 26% of cases [16] and 30″[33]; the optimum target should be less than 40″.[34] According to recent papers, the surgical cricothyrotomy should be faster than the Seldinger percutaneous technique.[35]

Percutaneous Cricothyrotomy

It has been since twenty years that many percutaneous cricothyrotomy sets, allowing introduction of an at least 4 mm ID cannula, have been designed and available on the market.

Whatever the set, all of them are based on airway identification as first step. An objective test is syringe aspiration, as described for simple tracheal puncture, followed by Seldinger guidewire introduction; subjective identification techniques are different from air aspiration and based on operators' "feeling" to insert an introducer in a empty channel followed by the cannula railroading over it, or on the visual identification of a spring mounted stylet movement.

The patient should be possibly supine, the head hyperextended; the operator's position, similarly to the surgical technique, is indifferent and variable, according to the operator's preferences in using a percutaneous cricothyrotomy set he should be preliminarily familiar with.

The cricothyroid membrane should be punctured in the midline and in the lower quadrant and the trachea possibly identified by free air aspiration through a liquid prefilled syringe. Using a Seldinger guidewire approach, the syringe is removed and a dedicated guidewire passed through the needle (or through a catheter over the needle) checking the possibility of a continuous, free and smooth "to and from" movement; when using such an approach, larynx immobilization can be interrupted after needle removal. After a no more than 0.5 cm skin incision is performed on both sides of guidewire, a dilator pre-mounted cannula is railroaded over the guidewire and inserted in a single maneuver. The dilator is finally removed and ventilation might be started. A large ID cannula allows adequate exhalation at a suggested respiratory rate of 10-12 min^{-1} [36], easy CO_2 detection and airways suction and the less used cuffed cannulas 6.0 mm ID (or more), while allowing a very effective either spontaneous or mechanical ventilation, are more difficult to insert in emergency.

An adult patient cannot spontaneously breathe through any cannula smaller than 4 mm ID. The 4 mm cannula doubles the normal inspiratory work of breathing while a 6 mm ID tube increases it by only 25% [37]; on the other hand the latter allows adequate insufflation and complete exhalation in about 4", with a 10-12 insufflations / min[-1] rate [38] and the possibility of effective tracheal aspiration.

Several manufacturers offer a variety of sets and cannula sizes with or without a cuff, with variable length ranging from 4 to 9 cm, outer diameter between 5 and 10 mm, inner diameter between 3.5 and 7.2 mm and different flange characteristics.

If considering as cut-off value for effective ventilation the 4 mm inner diameter, the Seldinger based kits commercially available with this diameter are represented by *MiniTrach II Seldinger*® (Portex-Smith) with 4.0 mm ID cannula (5.4 mm OD), the *Melker*® (Cook) with 4.0 mm ID cannula (5.0 mm OD) and 6.0 mm ID (7.0 mm OD), also available in the cuffed version (5.0 mm or 6.0 mm ID). Whenever using an adequate size cannula, the percutaneous cricothyrotomy grants many advantages such an easier procedure if compared with surgical dissection and in any case more familiar to the anesthesiologist. Seldinger versions of *MiniTrach*® and *Melker*® cricothyrotomy set are probably more time consuming than surgical procedure, but undoubtfully safer because they allow an air aspiration test, to check the free movement of the guide wire and to railroad the cannula on the guide wire without any need to immobilize the larynx.

MiniTrach II® (Portex-Smith), providing the same cannula than the Seldinger set and CPK® (Portex-Smith) available with 6.0 mm ID–9.0 mm OD are among non Seldinger based percutaneous cricothyrotomy sets. The most popular is the *Mini-Trach*, designed many years ago for tracheal aspiration in cases of sputum retention, but now a days largely used in emergency area; it is based on a blind insertion of a metal curved stylet-introducer after a small incision of both skin and crico-thyroideal membrane. The rigid blue stylet is easy to introduce in the stab membrane's incision only if the larynx is blocked between operator's fingers (see before)[39] and the feeling of correct insertion into the airway strictly depends on operator's sensitivity and experience.[40]

The diffusion of a specific set is not depending on safety only. A device may be very popular in a country because the insertion seems very rapid and faster when a prior incision is used,[41] and rarely used in another because the cannula's stiffness and because its insertion over a very sharp large needle seems to be potentially dangerous.

COMPLICATIONS

In emergency setting, all percutaneous techniques show the same complications high rate (procedural failure, posterior false route, pneumothorax, multiple attempts, severe bleeding) of surgical cricothyrotomy.[29] The complications rate incidence reported in the past[10] for 77 emergency cricothyrotomies in 8 years was:

- Wrong position: 12%
- Duration > three minutes: 8%
- Impossible positioning: 4%
- Hemorrhage: 6.5%
- Cartilage fracture and dysphonia (6.0 mm ID cannula): 1,5%

Other studies also describe:
- False route
- Esophageal perforation
- Intra and postoperative hemorrhage
- Laryngeal lesions
- Dysphonia and sore throat
- Subglottic stenosis
- Bronchial intubation
- Gastric aspiration
- Inferior laryngeal nerve lesion

LEARNING AND TRAINING

The failed intubation and the need for subsequent cricothyrotomy is a rarity, but most practitioners are unfamiliar with this life-saving technique. All emergency airway access techniques are potentially dangerous and present a high complication rate, especially if performed by unskilled personnel.[20] Training is very similarly the most difficult problem to solve in cricothyrotomy because a formal training on a regular basis is rarely done in most hospitals,[36] and even more rarely in terms of mandatory update requiring registrars training on both surgical cricothyrotomy and TTJV.[42]

The possibility to perform it on the consenting anesthetized patient scheduled for laryngectomy is frustrated by the increasingly reduction of this kind of radical surgery, and similarly the use of frozen pig's larynx has many practical disadvantages and organizing difficulties.

On the other hand, at least four possibilities for training still exist:
a. Cadavers about to undergo a medico-legal postmortem examination, after relatives consent.
b. ICU patients who need a temporary cricothyrotomy.
c. Self-education, achieved with hands-on courses on isolated trachea.
d. Dummies (*Bill II*® and *Frova Crico Trainer*® (Fig. 5.6) or similar products).

Cricothyrotomy is one of the procedures recommended by Italian difficult airway management guidelines [6] which consider mandatory the need to develop experience with such a procedure, leaving operators free to choose between tracheal puncture or cricothyrotomy while suggesting the use of Seldinger cricothyrotomy techniques with a cannula inner diameter equal or larger than the critical cut-off value of 4 mm.

Basal training should also consider continuous refreshments, considering that, similarly to other procedures, the manual dexterity for a rapid performance is gradually lost.

Comfortably, a mannequin study by Wong and coworkers[40] indicates in 5 attempts the number of procedures to obtain the minimal experience level with percutaneous cricothyrotomy, leading to the ability of a Seldinger procedure performance in less than 40".

The effect of SIAARTI recommendations [6] and training seems very good and would be interesting to be studied in the future, similarly to ASA Closed Claims Analysis Project [20], considering the increase of operatory theaters equipped with devices for difficult airway management,[43] even if equipment for percutaneous emergency tracheal access are still very rarely available in emergency departments, similarly to UK.[44]

CONCLUSIONS

The key point when speaking about cricothyrotomy is the development of familiarity with an easy to use device, allowing safe airway identification and providing an adequate diameter to provide both emergency oxygenation and ventilation. What really saves patient's life, indeed, is the physician or the paramedic (not in Italy today) knowing when to use emergency tracheal access and able to perform it before irreversible anoxic brain damage occurs. Preferred technique and device are important in conditioning maneuver's rapidity and efficiency, but the right time-choice for performing an emergency cricothyrotomy remains even more important, and it can only come from skilled

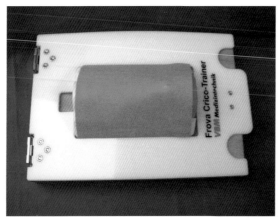

Fig. 5.6: Frova Crico Trainer

practice and from a clear mental and behavioral algorithm maintained with a repeated and constant practice.

Endotracheal tubes and cannulas used for cricothyrotomy might be either cuffed or uncuffed, but in any case they should offer an inner diameter larger than the critical one (4.0 – 4.5 mm) identified by Dworkin [36], avoiding in the meantime too larger diameters, which might represent a wrong choice in emergency setting for the previously described anatomical implications.

Simple tracheal puncture with small bore cannulas connected to low pressure gas sources is unable to deliver sufficient flow and provide adequate ventilation (CO_2 exhalation), but only provides one-way oxygen delivery and apneic oxygenation, remaining conditioned by the use of an adequate insufflation pressure; large diameter cuffed cannulas cannot be left in place for more than 24–48 hours, otherwise cricoideal or vocal cords injuries will appear. Between the two extremes, a large number of intermediate choices are available: a transtracheal approach using a cannula whose inner diameter is larger than the critical one and lower than 8 mm outer diameter allows adequate both manual and mechanical ventilation [45], this results being possible with either conventional open surgery or with percutaneous approach.

Emergency cricothyrotomy is a life saving procedure with a not low complication rate. There is almost no literature comparing different techniques, and this might be explained with the relatively rare performance of this procedure, which always occurs in urgent circumstances.

Anesthesia departments must select a cricothyrotomy device, and it must be available in operating theaters as well as in ICU, emergency unit, and first help portable bags. Success with its use is determined not only by its design but by familiarity with the set. There should be greater emphasis in the teaching hospitals about the matter that the difficult intubation algorithm should be both well taught and optimally learned.

Definitively, the incidence of CV-CI scenario requiring emergency airway access is felt to be too low for adequate training; this fact is misleading because we have to remember that all anesthesiologists have the probability to be called on to perform an invasive airway at some point in their career.

REFERENCES

1. Ward CF. Can't ventilate, can't intubate: What now? Seminars in Anestesia Perioperative Medicine and Pain. 2000;19:204-15.
2. Brantigan CO, Grow JB. Cicothyroidotomy: Elective use in respiratory problems requiring tracheostomy. J Thorac Cardiovas Surg 1976;71:72-81.
3. Brantigan CO, Grow JB. Cricothyroidotomy revisited again. Ear Nose Throat J 1980;59:26-38.
4. Henderson JJ, Popat MT, et al. Difficult Airway Society guidelines for management of the unanticipated difficult intubation. Anaesthesia 2004;59:675-94.
5. ASA Task Force on Management of the Difficult Airway. Practice guidelines for management of the difficult airway: An updated report by the American Society of Anesthesiologists Task Force on Management of the Difficult Airway. Anesthesiology 2003;98:1269-77.
6. Frova G (coordinator). SIAARTI Guidelines. Difficult intubation and management of difficult airways. Minerva Anestesiologica 1998;64:361-71.
7. Hachimi-Idrissi S, Huyghens L. International Liaison Committee on Resuscitation (ILCOR). Advanced cardiac life support update: The new ILCOR cardiovascular resuscitation guidelines. International Liaison Committee on Resuscitation. Eur J Emerg Med 2002;9:193-202.
8. De Latorre F, Nolan J, Robertson C, et al. European Resuscitation Council Guidelines 2000 for Adult Advanced Life Support. A statement from the Advanced Life Support Working Group and approved by the Executive Committee of the European Resuscitation Council. Resuscitation 2001;48:211-21.
9. Boyce JR, Peters GE, et al. Preemptive vessel dilator cricothyrotomy aids in the management of upper airway obstruction. Can J Anaesth 2005;52:765-9.
10. Erlandson MJ, Clinton JE, et al. Cricothyrotomy in the emergency department revisited. J Emerg Med 1989;7:115-8.
11. Fortune JB, Judkins DG, et al. Efficacy of prehospital surgical cricothyrotomy in trauma patients. Journal of Trauma 1997;42:832-6
12. Mutzbauer TS, Munz R, et al. Emergency cricothyroidotomy-puncture or anatomical preparation? Peculiarities of two methods for emergency airway access

demonstrated in a cadaver model. Anaesthesist 2003; 52:304-10.

13. Scrase I, Woollard M. Needle vs surgical cricothyroidotomy: A short cut to effective ventilation. Anaesthesia 2006;61:962-74.

14. Frerk C, Frampton C. Cricothyroidotomy: Time for change. Editorial. Anaesthesia 2006;61:921-3.

15. Benumof JL. Management of the difficult adult airway. Anesthesiology 1991;75:1087-110.

16. Bair AE, Filbin MR, et al. The failed intubation attempt in the emergency department: Analysis of prevalence, rescue techniques, and personnel. J Emerg Med 2002; 23:131-40.

17. Braun U, Goldman K, et al. Airway management. Leitlinie der deutschen gesellschaft für anaestesiologie und intesivmedizin. Anaesthesiologie und Intensivmedizin 2004;45:302-6.

18. Vissers RJ, Bair AE. Surgical Airway techniques. In: Walls RM et al. Manual of Emergency Airway Management. 2nd edn, Lippincott, Williams and Wilkins. 2004;157-82.

19. Parmet Jl, Colonna Romano P, et al. The laryngeal mask airway reliably provides rescue ventilation in cases of unanticipated difficult tracheal intubation along with difficult mask ventilation. Anesth Analg 1998;87:661-5.

20. Peterson GN, Domino KB, et al. Management of the difficult airway. A closed Claims Analysis. Anesthesiology 2005;103:33-9.

21. Boon JM, Abrahams PH, et al. Cricothyroidotomy: A clinical anatomy review. Clinical Anatomy 2004;17: 478-86.

22. Joint Royal Colleges Ambulance Liaison Committee. Clinical Practice Guidelines for the UK Ambulance Service, 2004. Available online at http://www.asancep.org.uk/JRCALC/guidelines).

23. Ravussin P, Freeman J. A new transtracheal catheter for ventilation and resuscitation. Can Anaesth Soc J 1985; 32:60-6.

24. Ryder IG, Paoloni CC, Harle CC. Emergency transtracheal ventilation: Assessment of breathing system chosen by anaesthetists. Anaesthesia 1996;51:764-8.

25. Benumof JL, Scheller MS. The importance of transtracheal jet ventilation in the management of the difficult airway. Anesthesiology 1989;71:769-78.

26. Holmes J, Panacek EA, et al. Comparison of two cricothyroidotomy techniques: Standard method versus rapid-four-step technique. Ann Emerg Med 1998;32:442-7.

27. McGill J, Clinton JE. Cricothyrotomy in the emergency department. Ann Emerg Med 1982;11:361-4.

28. Gillespie MB, Eisele DW. Outcomes of emergency surgical airway procedures in a hospital-wide setting. Laryngoscope 1999;109:1766-9.

29. Chan TC, Wilke GM, et al. Comparison of wire-guided cricothyrotomy versus standard surgical cricothyrotomy technique. J Emerg Med 1999;17:957-62.

30. Helm M, Gries A, et al. Surgical approach in difficult airway management. Best Practice & Research Clinical Anaesthesiology 2005;19:623-40.

31. Gerling MC, Davis DP, et al. Effect of surgical cricothyroidotomy on the unstable cervical spine in a cadaver model of intubation. J Emerg Med 2001;20:1-5.

32. Breitmeier D, Schultz Y, et al. Koniotomieubungen an der Leiche-Erfaharungen in der Ausbildung mit Medizinstudenten, Anaesthesisten und Notarzten. Anaesthesiol Intensivmed Notfallmed Schmerzther 2004; 39:94-100.

33. Wong DT, Lai K et al. Cannot intubate-cannot ventilate and difficult intubation strategies: Results of a Canadian national survey. Anesth Analg 2005;100:1439-46.

34. Craven R, Vanner RG. Ventilation of a model lung using various cricothyrotomy devices. Anaesthesia 2004;59: 595-9.

35. Sulaiman L, Tighe SQM et al. Surgical vs wire-guided cricothyroidotomy: A randomized crossover study of cuffed and uncuffed tracheal tube insertion. Anaesthesia 2006;61:565-70.

36. Dworkin R, Benumof JL, et al. The effective tracheal diameter that causes air trapping during jet ventilation. J Cardiothorac Anesth 1990;4:731-6.

37. Mullins JB, Templer JW, et al. Airway resistance and work of breathing in tracheostomy tubes. Laryngoscope. 1993;103:1367-72.

38. Biro P, Moe KS. Emergency transtracheal jet ventilation in high grade airway obstruction. J Clin Anesth 1997; 9: 604-7.

39. Clancy MJ. A study of the performance of cricothyroidotomy on cadavers using the Minitrach II. Arch Emerg Medicine 1989;6:143-5.

40. Wong DT, Pradhu AJ, et al. What is the minimum training required for successful cricothyroidotomy? A study in mannequin. Anesthesiology 2003;98:349-53.

41. Benumof JL, Skerman JH. Transtracheal ventilation. In: Benumof JL (ed): Clinical Procedures in Anesthesia and Intensive Care. Philadelphia, PA, Lippincott 1992;195-209.

42. O'Connor D, Longhorn R et al. Emergency surgical airway training in Western Australia. Anaesthesia 2004; 59:915.

43. Raccomandazioni SIAARTI per il controllo delle vie aeree e la gestione della difficoltà. Questionario conoscitivo per la valutazione dell'impatto nelle strutture operative. Now available online at http://www. vieaereedifficili.org.

44. Davies P. A stab in the dark: Are you ready for needle cricothyrotomy? Injury 1999;30:659-62.

45. Vanner R. Emergency cricothyrotomy. Current Anaesthesia and Critical Care 2001;12:238-43.

Chapter 6

Ciaglia's Techniques of Percutaneous Dilational Tracheostomy

Rudolph Puana, Joseph L Nates, Sushil P Ambesh

INTRODUCTION

In 1985, several years after Shelden et al[1] and Toye and Weinstein [2] first laid the ground work for their original tracheostomy techniques, a thoracic surgeon named Pasquale Ciaglia published his experience with a technique he had developed using a progressive dilatation of the trachea with multiple dilators.[3] Ciaglia's technique was based on the percutaneous nephrostomy procedure using the Amplatz kit[4,5] as well as years of surgical experience performing cricothyroidostomies as described by Brantigan and Grow.[6] The latter surgical approach had led to the development of a technique he called the fingertip sub-cricoid mini-tracheostomy.[5,7] The percutaneous dilational tracheostomy (PDT) gained immediate acceptance. The PDT rapidly spread world wide largely due to a few key factors: The ease and speed of insertion, decreased mortality and morbidity in relation to the surgical approach, and the overall decreased cost due to it safety and logistical advantages of not needing to transport patients to the operating room for the procedure.[8]

The original Ciaglia's PDT technique was commercially marketed using a kit manufactured by COOK® Critical Care, Bloomington, IN. Due to its popularity many manufacturers imitated Ciaglia's kit. These imitations have been associated with multiple problems such as: Using straight dilators instead of Ciaglia's anatomically curved dilators leading to a higher risk of damage of the posterior wall of the trachea (e.g. laceration of mucosa, perforation of the wall with development of tracheoesophageal fistulas), higher risk of tracheal rings fractures by the necessary bending of the rings to advance the dilators inside the tracheal lumen.[9,10] Consequently, the morbidity associated with these modifications has been wrongly attributed to the Ciaglia's PDT technique. This has lead to the confusion of many practitioners that are not aware of the many differences among the new techniques and modified kits. All of these techniques and different kits carry their own inherent morbidity and mortality, and in our opinion the term PDT should not be used interchangeably when comparing groups in any percutaneous tracheostomy study.

MULTIPLE DILATATION TECHNIQUE

The PDT technique originally described in the 1980's included multiple sequentially larger dilators ranging from a size 12 to 28-French; however, the present commercially available kit manufactured by COOK® Critical Care contains hydrophilic coated dilators up to a size 36-French allowing tracheal cannula to be inserted into the trachea (Fig. 6.1).

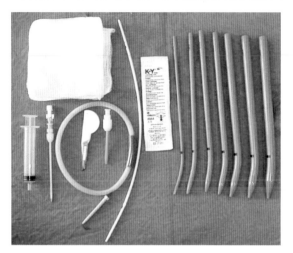

Fig. 6.1: Ciaglia's multiple dilators percutaneous tracheostomy kit (Cook Critical Care, Bloomington, IN, USA)

Although this technique is still widely used, but the multiple dilators kit is rapidly being replaced by a single, beveled and curved dilator, the Ciaglia's Blue Rhino, (CBR) kit in the United States and other countries. Though at many centers, Ciaglia's PDT technique is still practiced much as it was originally described, however, most clinicians recommend the use of fiberoptic bronchoscope for direct visualization of tracheal puncture, dilatation of tracheal stoma and to verify correct placement of tracheostomy tube.

The PDT is performed under general-relaxant anesthesia using 100% FiO_2 on controlled ventilation. The patient is positioned as for conventional surgical tracheostomy by placing a pillow or roll under the shoulders with the neck moderately extended to make the anatomical landmarks easily identifiable. Palpation of the trachea with identification of the cricoid cartilage, and the first, second, and third tracheal rings below the cricoid is (Fig. 6.2A) then performed for preparation of a sterile skin incision. The endotracheal tube (ETT) and oropharynx are suctioned clear. After identifying the proper level, 5-10 ml of 1% lidocaine with 1:200,000 epinephrine is infiltrated subcutaneously for local vasoconstriction.

- The respiratory therapist or anesthesiologist looking after the airway is asked to adjust the ventilator to compensate for desaturation, loss of sealing after deflating the ETT cuff, and adjusting the positive end-expiratory pressure (PEEP) as needed in preparation for the reposition of the tube. The cuff of the ETT is then deflated and pulled back to just below the vocal cords to avoid impalement of the ET tube or rupture of the cuff during the insertion of the tracheal puncture needle/cannula.

- A 1.5 cm vertical incision (most physicians we know including us, do a transverse incision for esthetic reasons) is made at the midline space below the cricoid cartilage and blunt dissection of pretracheal tissues is performed using hemostats to expose the pretracheal fascia.

- A 14-gauge introducer needle is then inserted in a posterio-caudad direction into the anterior trachea distal to the ETT with constant aspiration on the syringe between the first and second or second and third tracheal cartilaginous rings. Needle confirmation within the lumen of the trachea, and not impaled within the ETT, was done blindly when first described. Today, it is recommended to perform this step using direct fiberoptic bronchoscopic visualization. The successful introduction of the needle into the trachea confirmed by air bubbles into the saline filled syringe (Fig. 6.2B) during aspiration. On blind insertion of the introducer needle distal to the ETT is confirmed by rotation of the tube or moving the tube back and forth 1 cm without movement of the introducer needle; if movement of the needle occurs with the ETT rotation the needle is removed, the ETT is withdrawn a little more, and a new puncture is necessary.

- Once the cannula is in the correct position, a flexible 0.052 inch J tipped-wire is then inserted into the tracheal lumen (Fig. 6.2C).

- The cannula is then withdrawn, leaving the guide-wire *in situ*. A well-lubricated initial dilation is then performed with a short 11FG dilator; then for added firmness and stability, an 8 French Teflon guiding catheter with a safety ridge (to avoid damage to the posterior wall of the trachea during the manipulation of the dilators inside the trachea) is then advanced over the guide-wire (Fig. 6.2D).

• With the guide-wire still in place, the access site into the trachea is serially dilated by inserting up to six dilators ranging from 12 FG to 36 FG over the reinforced guide-wire set up (Fig. 6.3A). It is very important to properly align the dilator on the guide wire-guiding catheter assembly, position the proximal end of the dilator at the single positioning mark on the guiding

catheter. This will assure that the distal tip of the dilator is properly positioned at the safety ridge on the guiding catheter to prevent possible trauma to the posterior tracheal wall during introduction. Advance and pull back the dilating assembly several times, to perform effective dilatation of tracheal access point. The tracheostomy tube mounted on the corresponding size dilator is then threaded over the guide wire-guide catheter assembly, and introduced in to the tracheal stoma (Fig. 6.3B). The introducer and the guide wire-guide catheter are removed. The tracheostomy tube flanges are then secured with suture or ties around the neck.

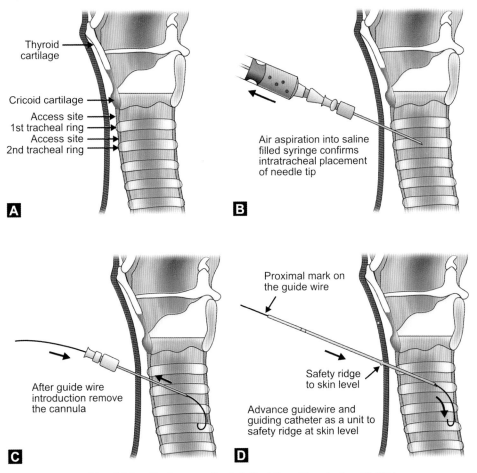

Figs 6.2A to D: *Courtesy:* Cook Critical Care Bloomington, IN, USA

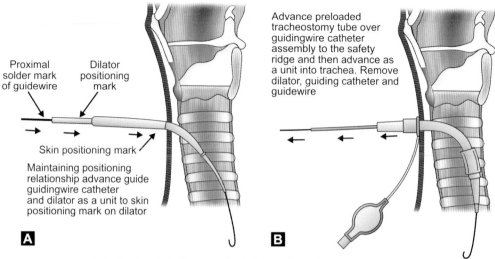

Proximal solder mark of guidewire

Dilator positioning mark

Skin positioning mark

Maintaining positioning relationship advance guide guidingwire catheter and dilator as a unit to skin positioning mark on dilator

Advance preloaded tracheostomy tube over guidingwire catheter assembly to the safety ridge and then advance as a unit into trachea. Remove dilator, guiding catheter and guidewire

A

B

Figs 6.3A and B: *Courtesy:* Cook Critical Care Bloomington, IN, USA

- It is better to slightly overdilate the tracheal stoma to allow easy passage of cuff portion of the appropriate size tracheostomy tube. For insertion of various tracheostomy tube sizes the recommended stoma dilation is as follows: For 6 mm (inner diameter) 24 FG, 7 mm (28 FG), 8 mm (32 FG) and for 9 mm (36 FG) dilation is required.
- Position of tracheostomy is then confirmed by end tidal CO_2 and/or direct bronchial visualization with a fiber optic bronchoscope.

The Single Tapered Dilator Technique The "Blue Rhino®"

In 1999, Ciaglia modified his own original technique by replacing the multiple dilators with a single tapered dilator "Blue Rhino®" (COOK® Critical Care, Bloomington, IN) (Fig. 6.4A). An imitation of the CBR is manufactured by Portex Ltd, UK where the main Rhino dilator is of white color (Fig. 6.4B). The single dilator has the advantage of not requiring a change in dilator, thereby reducing tidal volume loss until the tracheostomy tube is ready to be inserted.

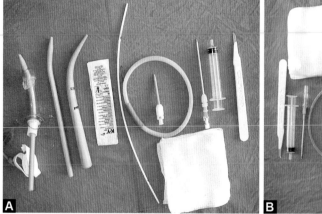
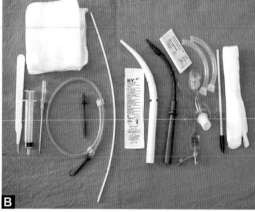

A

B

Figs 6.4A and B: (A) Ciaglia Blue Rhino percutaneous tracheostomy kit with tracheostomy tube and introducer (Cook Critical Care, IN, USA); **(B)** Portex percutaneous dilational tracheostomy kit with single stage dilator (similar to CBR) with blue line ultra tracheostomy tube and introducer (Portex Ltd. CT21 6JL, UK)

In the Ciaglia's Blue Rhino method, the technique is basically the same until the insertion of the guide-wire.[11] The EZ-pass hydrophilic coating on the CBR is activated by immersing the distal end in sterile water or saline. Advance the CBR dilator and the guiding catheter as a unit over the guide wire while maintaining the guide wire *in situ*. The proximal end of the guiding catheter is aligned at the mark on the proximal portion of the guide wire.

Begin to dilate the entrance site by advancing the guiding catheter and CBR dilator as a unit over the guide wire into the trachea to the skin level mark on the CBR dilator. Remove the CBR dilator, leaving the guide wire and guiding catheter assembly in position (Figs 6.5 and 6.6A and B).

Finally, the tracheostomy tube loaded over an appropriate and well-lubricated loading dilator (Fig. 6.7) is inserted through the tracheal stoma. The loading dilator, the guide-wire, and the guiding catheter are then removed, leaving the tracheostomy tube *in situ* (Figs 6.8A to D).

Technical Considerations of Ciaglia's techniques

There are many technical considerations in achieving safe and efficient insertion using Ciaglia's multiple dilation technique.

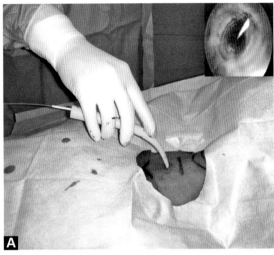

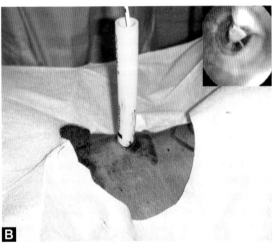

Figs 6.6A and B: (A) Formation of tracheal stoma by introducing the Ciaglia Blue Rhino over the guide wire and the guiding catheter (white). In inset: **(B)** Bronchoscopic visualization of guiding catheter and blue rhino inside the tracheal lumen

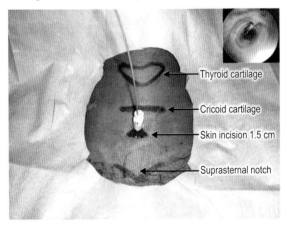

Fig. 6.5: Anatomical landmarks, 1.5 cm horizontal skin incision, guidewire and initial dilator *in situ*. (Inset) tip of the initial dilator over guide wire seen in tracheal lumen bronchoscopically

- First and foremost, patient selection plays a fundamental role in this process. The technique is not recommended for emergency airway access, in pediatric patients, or any patients with anatomical variations that preclude correct placement. Patients where landmarks are not identifiable should be taken to the operating room for an open surgical procedure.[12,13]

- Secondly, the operators need to be properly trained in the technique, have previous

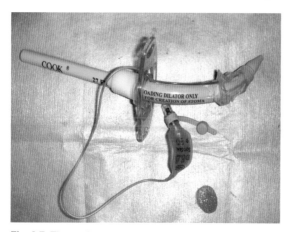

Fig. 6.7: The tracheostomy tube (8.5 mm ID) is kept ready on a loading dilator; tracheal cuff deflated and lubricated

experience with the Seldinger's technique, and had the dexterity required for surgical procedures that demand it; like in the case of airway surgery. Although the technique is simple, there are many details that are important procedurally to avoid fracturing the tracheal rings, injuring the posterior tracheal wall, lacerating the mucosa, or creating tracheoesophageal fistulas (e.g. proper angle of dilator insertion, positioning of the Teflon catheter, and use of the safety ridge).

- Thirdly, although two authors of this chapter (JLN & SPA) have performed PDTs in patients with PEEP pressures up to 20 cm H_2O without

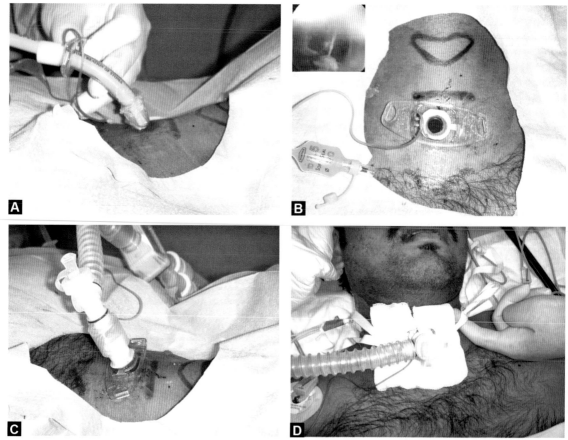

Figs 6.8A to D: (A) Introduction of tracheostomy tube **(B)** trachesotomy tube *in situ* and tracheal cuff inflated with air. Positioning of the tube in tracheal lumen is confirmed by seeing carina bronchoscopically. (Inset). **(C and D)** Tracheostomy tube connected with breathing circuit and secured with the ties around the neck

complications, it is recommended that mechanically ventilated patients with high peak airway pressures should be postponed until peak pressures can be weaned to avoid hypoxemia during the period in which PEEP is lost.

• Fourthly, the kit used may influence the outcome of the procedure as well as the individual that is handling the airway. Lack of an experienced anesthesiologist could potentially increase the complications associated with airway manipulation and anesthesia (e.g. desaturation, loss of airway control, hypotension, cardiac arrhythmias, and even cardiac arrest). If not properly taken in consideration, co-morbidities ranging from morbid obesity to coagulopathies may play a role in patient outcome when deciding to perform this procedure.

Compared to other percutaneous tracheostomy kits, the Ciaglia's kits made by COOK® Critical Care rank highest in authors' view. There are several key differences between these kits and other kits for the same and different techniques, such as the Fantoni's translaryngeal tracheostomy (TLT),[14] Frova's PercuTwist,[15] Griggs' guide-wire dilation forceps (GWDF),[16] Ambesh T-Dagger,[17] etc. Complications associated with the different kits and techniques include surgical time, bleeding, and performance variability among different skill groups.

CLINICAL CONSIDERATIONS AND COMPARISONS

Many advantages of Ciaglia's PDT technique have been shown in several studies.[7,18-21] One of the advantages of the Ciaglia's (Cook) kit, is the Teflon catheter that reinforces the guide-wire reducing kinking and para-tracheal placement of tracheostomy tube. Ciaglia's progressive dilation causes tamponade on tracheal tissue decreasing perioperative bleeding. Ciaglia's kit is simple and allows for a few quick individual dilations with average insertion time around 7 minutes.[18-21]

When comparing other percutaneous kits to Ciaglia's kit, each kit offers its own advantage and disadvantages. The Fantoni's percutaneous tracheostomy takes advantage of a retrograde translaryngeal approach and uses some of the same principles as Ciaglia's technique. Yet, due to the route of insertion it is otherwise very technically difficult for the novice operator. The Fantoni kit has 13 individual parts with over 14 separate steps for insertion. Despite its complexity, the Fantoni approach is one of the few techniques that have been successfully carried out on highly unstable patients,[22] infants and children.[23] Due to the less traumatic pressure on the anterior wall, it is ideal for patients with bleeding diathesis and goiters. The disadvantages are the complexity of the kit leading to the need of a very experienced operator, and the fact that bronchoscopy is essential. Another disadvantage is a significant apneic period during the retrograde pull-through. It makes this approach contraindicated in cases of difficult airways where exchanging endotracheal tubes is not safe, in patients with significant acidosis or head injury patients where pCO_2 levels must be strictly maintained.

Ciaglia's newer single dilation method as compared to his multiple dilator technique is thought to have many of the same attributes of the original Cook Ciaglia multiple dilator kit. This Ciaglia's technique uses a simpler kit with less parts and dilation attempts making the CBR a faster and even more attractive technique than the multiple dilators. The reduced number of dilatations performed makes patients less exposed to the risk of posterior wall laceration. Despite the report by Byhahn where Ciaglia's PDT with multiple dilators performed better than the CBR in terms of lesser incidence of tracheal cartilage rupture (2/25 vs 9/25),[24] the latter seems to be rapidly replacing the old Ciaglia's technique in America. Clinically speaking, it is felt by this author (JLN), that the Blue Rhino possibly has the same bleeding rates as Ciaglia's multiple dilator technique and has fewer steps which consequently take less time. The CBR relies on the classic Ciaglia approach with an anatomically curved dilator and very few steps.

Being that the advent of the CBR kit is fairly new, there are no large randomized studies comparing this technique. In a single randomized, observational clinical trial of elective percutaneous tracheostomy (n = 70). Byhahn compared two single-dilator percutaneous tracheostomy techniques, the CBR (n = 35) and the new PercuTwist technique (n = 35), another single dilator method.[25] The CBR out performed the PercuTwist. In this study, there were two incidences of posterior tracheal wall injury from PercuTwist dilatation. Stoma dilation was successful with the respective device in all patients. While subsequent tracheostomy cannula insertion was uneventful in all but one patient undergoing the Blue Rhino technique, it was difficult or even impossible in eight patients who underwent PercuTwist tracheostomy. Regarding serious and intermediate procedural-related complications, two cases of posterior tracheal wall injury occurred with the PercuTwist technique. No serious or intermediate complications were noted during Blue Rhino tracheostomy. Conclusions could not be made due to the small numbers in the study, but experience was said to be a major contributor.

In a preliminary study, Luna Azoulay et al [26] in a retrospective study of endoscopically guided percutaneous tracheostomy, CBR (n = 28), PercuTwist (n = 2), observed no intraoperative or early postoperative complications in twenty-two (73.3%) patients. Eight complications were observed, half preoperative and half early postoperative. Three patients (10%) had minor bleeding. The most important complication was intraoperative appearance of a tracheoesophageal fistula with the CBR. They concluded that the PDT is a safe and valid alternative procedure to surgical tracheostomy, however, though initially performed by intensivists, it should be part of the ENT/head and neck surgeon's repertory as the upper airway specialist.

Divisi et al [27] compared the operative technique and complications of the TLT with those of the CBR; TLT in 350 and CBR in 120 adult critically ill patients. The CBR tracheostomy was noted to have a cost-benefit advantage over TLT. The CBR tracheostomy took less time to perform and had fewer complications than TLT, because the technique was simpler.

In a prospective, randomized, comparative study of CBR versus T-Dagger PDT kits, Ambesh et al [28] noticed significant increase in peak airway pressure (PAP) when the patient were on controlled ventilation while the CBR was *in situ*. The T-dagger scored better in this regard as the rise in PAP was not significant. Further, the CBR was associated with more tracheal cartilaginous ring fracture.

Romero and coworkers[29] have evaluated the safety of performing percutaneous tracheostomy (PT) using the CBR technique with fiberoptic bronchoscopy assistance in patients with prolonged mechanical ventilation in ICU. In a prospective study 100 consecutive patients aged 62 ± 16 years (38 women) were subjected to PT. Demographic variables, APACHE II, days of mechanical ventilation before PT, operative and postoperative complications were recorded. Eight patients (8%) had operative complications. One had an episode of transitory desaturation, one had a transitory hypotension related to sedation and six had mild bleeding not requiring transfusion. No patient required conversion to surgical tracheostomy. Four patients (4%) presented postoperative complications. Two had a mild and transitory bleeding of the ostomy and two had a displacement of the cannula. No other complications were observed. The study concluded that the PT using the CBR technique under fibreoptic bronchoscopy assistance is a safe procedure and can be performed in the ICU by trained intensivists.

CONCLUSION

In summary, the Ciaglia techniques are among the safest and most popular percutaneous techniques in use. The PDT has had a major impact in patient care since Ciaglia described it in 1985, and has become the Gold Standard by which all the other percutaneous techniques are measured. Pasquale Ciaglia's extensive research in the development of this device using animal models, human trials, and research cohorts are unparalleled among the other techniques. Although Ciaglia died before finishing his latest innovation to the PDT technique, an inflatable dilator, he left behind an enormous and precious legacy.

REFERENCES

1. Sheldon CH, Pudenz RH, Freshwater DB, Crue BL. A new method for tracheotomy. J Neurosurg 1957;12: 428-31.
2. Toye FJ, Weinstein JD. A percutaneous tracheostomy device. Surgery 1969;65:384-9.
3. Ciaglia P, Firsching R, Syniec C. Elective percutaneous dilatational tracheostomy: A new simple bedside procedure; preliminary report. Chest 1985;87:715-9.
4. Nates JL, Cooper DJ, Myles PS, Scheinkestel CD, Tuxen DV. Percutaneous tracheostomy in critically ill patients: A prospective, randomized comparison of two techniques. Crit Care Med 2000;28(11):3734-9.
5. Ciaglia P, Firshing R, Syniec C. Elective percutaneous dilational tracheostomy: A new simple bedside procedure-Preliminary report. Chest 1985;87:715-9.
6. Brantigan CO, Grow JB Sr. Cricothyroidotomy: elective use in respiratory problems requiring tracheotomy. J Thorac Cardiovasc Surg 1976;71:72-81.
7. Nates JL, Anderson MB, Cooper DJ. Percutaneous dilational tracheostomy: A clinical study evaluating two systems. Anaesth Intensive Care 1997;25:194-5.
8. Griggs WM, Myburgh JA, Worthley LI. A prospective comparison of a percutaneous tracheostomy technique with standard surgical tracheostomy. Intensive Care Med 1991;17:261-3.
9. Nates JL, Marx D, Cocanour C, et al. Percutaneous tracheostomy, with the SIMS kit. Crit Care Med 1999; 27:735.
10. Trottier SJ, Ritter S, Lakshmanan R, Sakabu SA, Troop BR. Percutaneous tracheostomy tube obstruction warning. Chest 2002;122:1377-81.
11. Ambesh SP, Swanevelder JL. Percutaneous dilational tracheostomy. Ann Card Anaesth 2004;7:77-85.
12. Friedman Y. Indications, timing, technique, and complications of tracheostomy in the critically ill. Curr Opin Crit Care 1996;2:47-53.
13. Durbin CG. Indications for and timing of tracheostomy. Respir Care 2005;50:483-7.
14. Fantoni A, Ripamonti D. A non-derivative, non-surgical tracheostomy: the translaryngeal method. Intensive Care Med 1997;23:386-92.
15. Frova G, Quintel M. A new simple method for percutaneous tracheostomy: Controlled rotating dilation. A preliminary report. Intensive Care Med 2002;28: 299-303.
16. Griggs WM, Worthley LIG, Gilligan JE, Thomas PD, Myburg JA. A simple percutaneous tracheostomy technique. Surg Gynecol Obstet 1990;170:543-5.
17. Ambesh SP, Tripathi M, Pandey CK, Pant KC, Singh PK. Clinical evaluation of the "T-Dagger": A new bedside percutaneous dilational tracheostomy device. Anaesthesia 2005;60:708-11.
18. Añón JM, Gomez-Tello V, de Paz V, et al. Percutaneous dilational tracheostomy: Comparison of Ciaglia and Griggs systems. Crit Care Med 1999;27:A70.
19. Ambesh SP, Percutaneous dilational tracheostomy: The Ciaglia method versus the Portex method. Anesth Analg 1998;87-556-61.
20. Ambesh SP, Pandey CK, Srivastava S, Agarwal A, Singh DK. Percutaneous tracheostomy with single dilatation technique: A prospective, randomized comparison of Ciaglia blue rhino versus Griggs guidewire dilating forceps. Anesth Analg 2002;95:1739-45.
21. Nates JL, Cooper DJ, Myles PS, Scheinkestel CD, Tuxen DV. Percutaneous tracheostomy in critically ill patients: a prospective, randomized comparison of two techniques. Crit Care Med 2000;28:3734-9.
22. Byhahn C, Lischke V, Westphal K. Translaryngeal tracheostomy in highly unstable patients. Anaesthesia 2000;55:678-82.
23. Fantoni A, Ripamonti D. Tracheostomy in pediatrics patients. Minerva Anestesiol 2002;68:433-42.
24. Byhahn C, Wilke HJ, Halbig S, Lischke V, Westphal K. Percutaneous tracheostomy: Ciaglia Blue Rhino versus the basic Ciaglia technique of percutaneous dilational tracheostomy. Anesth Analg 2000;91:882-6.
25. Byhahn C, Westphal K, Meininger D, Gurke B, Kessler P, Lischke V. Single-dilator percutaneous tracheostomy: a comparison of PercuTwist and Ciaglia Blue Rhino techniques. Intensive Care Med 2002;28:1262-6.
26. Luna Azoulay B, Béquignon A, Babin E, Moreau S. Preliminary results of percutaneous tracheotomies. Ann Otolaryngol Chir Cervicofac 2009; May 21.

27. Divisi D, Altamura G, Di Tommaso S, Di Leonardo G, Rosa E, De Sanctis C, Crisci R. Fantoni translaryngeal tracheostomy versus Ciaglia blue rhino percutaneous tracheostomy: A retrospective comparison. Surg Today 2009;39:387-92.

28. Ambesh SP, Pandey CK, Tripathi M, Pant KC, Singh PK. Formation of bedside percutaneous tracheostomy with the T-Dagger: A prospective randomized and comparative evaluation with the Ciaglia Blue Rhino. Anesthesiology 2005;103:A316.

29. Romero P C, Cornejo R R, Ruiz C M, Gálvez A R, Llanos V O, Tobar A E, Larrondo G J, Castro O J. Fiberoptic bronchoscopy assisted percutaneous tracheostomy: Report of 100 patients. Rev Med Chil 2008;136:1113-20.

Chapter 7

Griggs' Technique of Percutaneous Dilational Tracheostomy

Sushil P Ambesh

In 1985 Ciaglia et al published a sequential dilatation technique to form percutaneous tracheostomy (PCT).[1] This technique became quite popular and by the end of 1980s it reached to many hospitals of United States of America, Europe and Australia. Dr Griggs, a consultant at Royal Adelaide Hospital, Adelaide, Australia and his colleagues postulated that the surgical technique of blunt dissection may create same type of tracheal stoma if a pair of forceps could be placed in the correct position.[2] The concept of using a guidewire to place such forceps correctly seemed reasonable. After some initial unsuccessful attempts, a pair of guidewire dilating forceps (GWDF) was developed by Dr Griggs with the help of his father, a formally trained mechanical engineer. The GWDF is like a grooved Howard Kelly forceps, in which the guidewire passes through a hole in the tip of the closed forceps, thus leading them in the right direction. Spreading the forceps by pulling the handles apart dilates the trachea over the guidewire in the right direction.

First clinical trial was done at Royal Adelaide Hospital and results were published.[3] The initial technique that was performed in 153 patients (108 males and 45 females) involved the insertion of a Seldinger guide wire between the cricoid and first tracheal ring or between two lower tracheal rings. The GWDF were advanced along the wire into the trachea and opened to split the tracheal membrane to the diameter of tracheostomy. An appropriately sized tracheostomy tube and trocar were then inserted over the guide wire and advanced into the trachea. General anesthesia was used in 150 patients and local anesthesia was used in 3 patients. The procedure, done electively, was completed in 3-8 minutes. There was no mortality. Hemorrhage was the only complication and that occurred in 2 patients.

Presently, the kit is being manufactured for clinical use by SIMS, Portex Ltd, Hythe, Kent, UK (Fig. 7.1A). When forceps are closed, a tunnel formed at the tip will allow the guide wire to pass through the forceps' blades (Fig. 7.1B).

Since then a number of prospective and controlled studies have been published[4-10] and procedural steps have been defined in great details.

ANESTHESIA

- General anesthesia and muscle relaxation with the type and dosage of medications dictated by the clinical needs of the patient.
- Place the patient on 100% oxygen throughout the procedure.

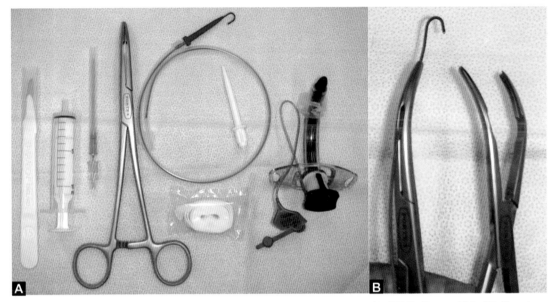

Figs 7.1A and B: (A) Various parts of Griggs' percutaneous tracheostomy kit (SIMS; Portex, UK); **(B)** Showing passage of the guide wire (in closed position) and grooves in the forceps (open)

- Hyperextend the patient's neck if no contraindications exist. Before preparation of the surgical area begins, withdrawal of the endotracheal tube under direct vision of bronchoscope is recommended to place the balloon just under the vocal cords. The respiratory therapist then protects the tube against any further movement during the procedure.
- Infiltrate the incision site with a solution (5-10 ml) of 1-2% lignocaine with 1:100,000 adrenaline.

The neck is cleansed with antiseptic solution and properly draped. The neck is palpated, and the cricoid cartilage is identified. The skin below this level is anesthetized by infiltrating 5-10 ml of 1% lignocaine with 1:100,000 adrenaline solution. A 1.5 to 2 cm transverse skin incision is made at midline directly over the preselected site (Fig. 7.2), followed by a blunt dissection using a curved forceps or the GWDF itself. The left middle finger and thumb are used to secure the lateral edges of the trachea, while the index finger is used to locate the intercartilagenous area previously selected.

A 14-gauge introducer needle with cannula connected to a saline filled syringe held by the right hand, is inserted in the midline of the trachea and advanced into the tracheal lumen under continuous aspiration by withdrawing the plunger of the attached syringe. The needle is directed to pass between the first and second or second and third tracheal rings, rather than between the cricoid and the first tracheal ring. The intratracheal needle placement is guided by direct bronchoscopic visualization (Fig. 7.3) and confirmed by free aspiration of air in the attached saline filled syringe. As soon as air begins to bubble into the syringe, the outer plastic cannula is advanced into the lumen of the trachea and the introducer needle is removed. Many a times, tracheal secretion or mucous is aspirated in the syringe through correctly placed cannula in tracheal lumen.

A J-tipped guide wire is placed via the Seldinger technique and the plastic cannula is removed. Now, the formation of tracheal stoma is initiated by passing a 14 G well lubricated initial dilator through the anterior tracheal wall over the guidewire (Fig. 7.4).

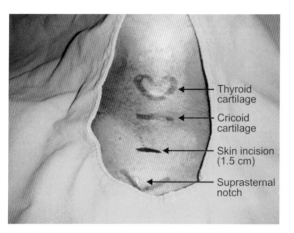

Fig. 7.2: Various anatomical landmarks and skin incision for percutaneous tracheostomy

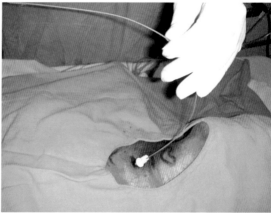

Fig. 7.4: Initial dilator passed over the guidewire in order to initiate stoma formation

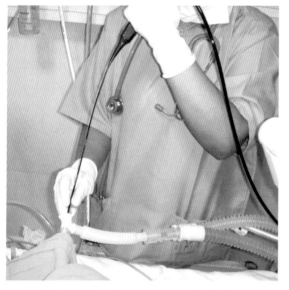

Fig. 7.3: Direct bronchoscopic visualization of tracheal puncture

The dilator is removed and the GWDF is passed (closed position) over the guidewire. The forceps are now advanced along the guidewire through the soft tissues of neck piercing the anterior tracheal wall and entering the tracheal lumen. The direction of the forceps is now changed by lifting the handles of GWDF towards the chin of the patient. The forceps are now opened by pulling the handles apart with both hands keeping strict vigil on the tracheal stoma for appropriate dilatation (Figs 7.5A to D). Never open the forceps in the position shown in Fig. 7.5B, as it may cause serious injuries to the posterior tracheal wall. The forceps are now removed in open position, leaving the guidewire *in situ*.

A two stage dilation procedure may also be used, opening the blades in front of the trachea first to dilate pretracheal tissues before inserting the guidewire. A previously prepared and well lubricated tracheostomy tube with its obturator is inserted over the guidewire and advanced into the tracheal lumen. The obturator and guidewire are removed, the cuff of the tracheostomy tube is inflated, and tracheostomy suction is done (Figs 7.6A and B).

An appropriate breathing circuit is connected. If there is subcutaneous bleeding that can be stopped by applying the external digital pressure and inflating the tracheal cuff. The tracheostomy tube is secured with the help of ribbon ties around the neck in such a way that it is not too loose or too tight, and that can be checked by inserting a finger beneath the ribbon ties (Fig. 7.7). Following confirmation of correct placement of tracheostomy tube the oropharyngeal suction is done, cuff deflated and ET tube is removed.

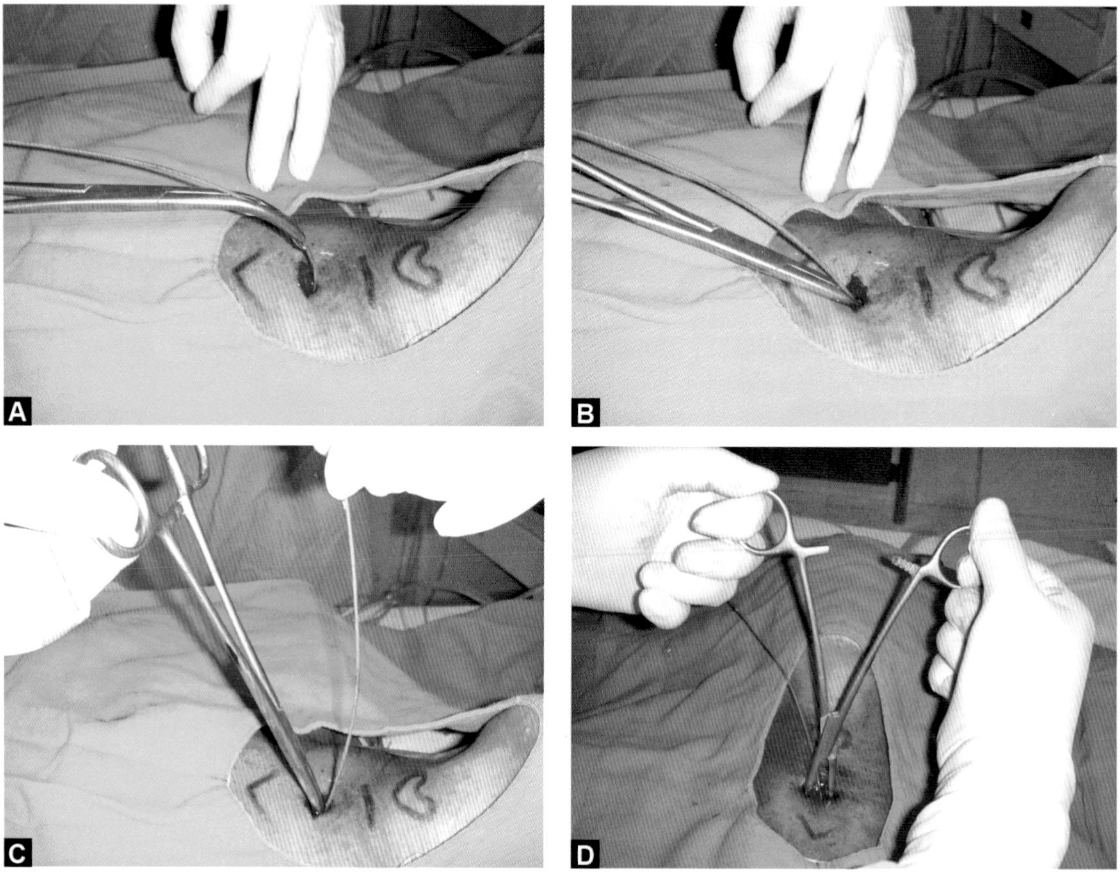

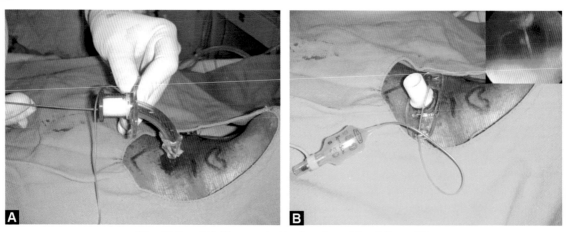

Figs 7.5A to D: Introduction of Griggs' forceps over the guidewire and formation of appropriate size of tracheal stoma

Figs 7.6A and B: Placement of tracheostomy tube (8.5 mm ID)

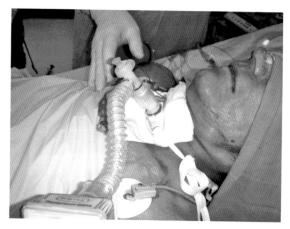

Fig. 7.7: Tracheostomy tube is secured with the ties around the neck

Bronchoscopic guidance to visualize tracheal puncture, the guidewire insertion and dilatation of tracheal stoma is optional but strongly recommended; especially for less-experienced operators.[11] A large number of paratracheal cannula insertions and pneumothoraces can be avoided if endoscopic monitoring is employed.[12,13] Bronchoscopic monitoring also allows patients with short, fat necks to undergo PCT. However, bronchoscopic guidance during PCT appears to be the most important factor responsible for the hypercapnea that develops during the procedure.[14] Therefore, bronchoscopic guidance should be limited to initial dilatation steps only.

Postoperative Details

- Air entry into the lungs is checked by chest auscultation and respiratory plethysmography.
- Excess secretions or blood should be suctioned to prevent a drop in oxygen saturation and to provide good bronchopulmonary hygiene.
- Everyday antiseptic wound care must be provided. A tracheostomy tube with an inner cannula facilitates care and hygiene and ensures added safety (due to easy removal) if obstruction from secretions occurs.
- In the event of accidental decannulation within 5-7 days of the procedure, the patient may need to be reintubated orally if the tracheostomy tube cannot be immediately reinserted because the tracheostomy tract is still relatively immature.

Follow-up

- Monitor the patient to prevent dislodgment of the tracheostomy tube.
- Deliver oxygen and/or mechanical ventilation as needed to maintain the patient's oxygen saturation and maintain appropriate ventilation.
- If using a cuffed tracheostomy tube, monitor cuff pressure carefully because prolonged inflation and/or over-inflation can lead to tracheal mucosal injury.
- Clean the inner cannula as much as needed to clear secretions at least once every 8 hours.
- Suction the trachea as needed.

The Griggs technique is very popular in Australia and outside of the United States. The advantages of this technique are, particularly in experienced hands, its speed and extreme simplicity. The procedure is very elegant and can be taught very rapidly. Airway patency can be achieved in less than 5 minutes with low complication rates. A number of prospective, controlled studies have compared Griggs' technique with Ciaglia's technique.

Van Heerden et al[15] reported no significant differences between the Ciaglia and Griggs PDTs. However, when analyzed by Nates et al,[16] there were 20% surgical complication rate with Griggs PDT (three bleeding, one infection, one paratracheal placement of tube among 25 patients) and a 6.5% complication rate with the Ciaglia PDT (two bleeding in 29 patients). Ambesh and Kaushik[4] also reported no significant difference between the two techniques, although the Griggs technique was faster (6.5 ± 3.5 mins vs 14 ± 5.5 mins) compared with the Ciaglia's multiple dilators PDT technique. In an another study, Ambesh et al[9] compared Griggs forceps with Ciaglia Blue Rhino (CBR) and have reported higher incidence of bleeding and inadequate or over formation of tracheal stoma with

Griggs forceps in majority of patients and attributed it to uncontrolled and unmeasured dilatation of tracheal stoma. Escarment et al[17] also reported under-dilatation of tracheal stoma in almost two-third of his patients on first attempt and required two or more attempts before tracheostomy tube could be inserted. This technique leads to increased tissue damage with an increased risk of bleeding and infection similar to the open surgical method unlike the Ciaglia technique causing a tamponade effect with its dilation. Nates et al[18] postulated that these surgical complications are probably due to uncontrolled dilatation with Griggs forceps.

Kluge et al[19] performed bedside percutaneous tracheostomy under bronchoscopy in 42 severely thrombocytopenic patients using Griggs' technique. The mean platelet count was $26.4 \pm 11.6 \times 10(9)$ cells/L. Before the procedure 40 patients received about six units of platelets transfusion. Twenty-two patients (52%) had an additional coagulopathy (activated partial thromboplastin time > 40 s; international normalized ratio > 1.5). PT was safely performed in all 42 patients. Only two (5%) patients developed major postprocedural bleeding complications that required suturing. Both of these patients had an elevated APTT due to heparin therapy. The authors concluded that when performed by experienced personnel, PT with bronchoscopic guidance has a low complication rate in patients with severe thrombocytopenia, provided that platelets are administered before hand. However, in order to minimize bleeding complications heparin infusions should be temporarily interrupted during the procedure.

Recently, Yuca et al[20] performed fiberoptic guided percutaneous dilational tracheostomy with GWDF in 52 critically ill patients. The duration of the GWDF technique was about 5 min. Intraoperative complications occurred in 10 (19.2%) patients: hemorrhage in three cases, puncture of the tracheal tube in two cases, difficult cannulation in two cases, difficult dilatation in one case, false passage in one case, and inadvertent extubation in one case. Postoperative complications occurred in three (5.7%) patients, stomal cellulitis in one case, subcutaneous emphysema in one case, and difficult recannulation in one case. The study concluded that fiberoptic bronchoscopy-assisted percutaneous dilatational tracheostomy by GWDF is a simple and fast technique for inserting a tracheal cannula.

REFERENCES

1. Ciaglia P, Firsching R, Syniec C. Elective percutaneous dilational tracheostomy. Chest 1985;87:715-9.
2. Griggs WM. Development of the Guide Wire Dilating Forceps (Griggs) technique. J Fur Anasthesie Intensvbehandlung 2006;3:13-4.
3. Griggs WM, Worthley LIG, Gilligan JE, Thomas PD, Myburg JA. A simple percutaneous tracheostomy technique. Surg Gynecol Obstet 1990;170:543-5.
4. Ambesh SP, Percutaneous dilational tracheostomy: The Ciaglia method versus the Portex method. Anesth Analg 1998;87-556-61.
5. Nates JL, Cooper DJ, Myles PS, Scheinkestel CD, Tuxen DV. Percutaneous tracheostomy in critically ill patients: A prospective, randomized comparison of two techniques. Crit Care Med 2000;28:3734-9.
6. Steele AP, Evans HW, Afaq MA, Robson JM, Dourado J, Tayar R, Stockwell MA. Long-term follow-up of Griggs percutaneous tracheostomy with spiral CT and questionnaire. Chest 2000;117:1430-3.
7. Byhahn C, Wilke HJ, Lischke V, Rinne T, Westphal K. Bedside percutaneous tracheostomy: Clinical comparison of Griggs and Fantoni techniques. World J Surg 2001;25:296-301.
8. Watters MPR, Thorne G, Cox CM, Monk CR. Tracheal rupture during percutaneous tracheostomy: Safety aspects of the Griggs method. Br J Anaesth 2000;84:671-2.
9. Ambesh SP, Pandey CK, Srivastava S, Agarwal A, Singh DK. Percutaneous tracheostomy with single dilatation technique: A prospective, randomized comparison of Ciaglia blue rhino versus Griggs guidewire dilating forceps. Anesth Analg 2002;95:1739-45.
10. Yuca K, Kati I, Tekin M, Yilmaz N, Tomak Y, Cankaya H. Fiber optic bronchoscopy assisted percutaneous dilataional tracheostomy by guidewire dilating forceps in intensive care unit patients. J Otolaryngol Head Neck Surg 2008;37:76-80.
11. Kost KM. Endoscopic percutaneous dilatational tracheotomy: A prospective evaluation of 500 consecutive cases. Laryngoscope Oct 2005;115:1-30.

12. Marelli D, Paul A, Manolidis S, et al. Endoscopic guided percutaneous tracheostomy: Early results of a consecutive trial. J Trauma 1990;30:433-5.

13. Fernandez L, Norwood S, Roettger R, Gass D, Wilkins H 3rd. Bedside percutaneous tracheostomy with bronchoscopic guidance in critically ill patients. Arch Surg 1996;131:129-32.

14. Reilly PM, Anderson HL, Singh RF, Schwab CW, Barlett RH. Occult hypercarbia: An unrecognised phenomenon during percutaneous endoscopic tracheostomy. Chest 1995;107:1760-3.

15. Van Heerden PV, Webb SA, Power BM, et al. Percutaneous dilational tracheostomy: A clinical study evaluating two systems. Anaesth Intensive Care 1996;24:56-9.

16. Nates JL, Anderson MB, Cooper DJ. Percutaneous dilational tracheostomy: A clinical study evaluating two systems. Anesth Analg 1997;25:194-5.

17. Escarment J, Suppini A, Sallaberry M, Kaiser E, Cantais E, Palmier B, Quinot JF. Percutaneous tracheostomy by forceps dilation. Report of 162 cases. Anaesthesia 2000; 55:125-30.

18. Nates JL, Cooper DJ, Myles PS, Scheinkestel CD, Tuxen DV. Percutaneous tracheostomy in critically ill patients: A prospective randomized comparison of two techniques. Crit Care Med 2000;28:3734-9.

19. Kluge S, Meyer A, Kühnelt P, Baumann HJ, Kreymann G. Percutaneous tracheostomy is safe in patients with severe thrombocytopenia. Chest 2004;126:547-51.

20. Yuca K, Kati I, Tekin M, Yilmaz N, Tomak Y, Cankaya H. Fiberoptic bronchoscopy-assisted percutaneous dilatational tracheostomy by guidewire dilating forceps in intensive care unit patients. J Otolaryngol Head Neck Surg 2008;37:76-80.

Chapter 8

Frova's PercuTwist Percutaneous Dilational Tracheostomy

Giulio Frova, Massimiliano Sorbello

INTRODUCTION

Tracheostomy, an invasive procedure largely performed in ICU, is aimed to obtain a direct access to the airway. On the terminological point of view the terms *tracheotomy* and *tracheostomy* are used indifferently as synonyms.[1] If compared with translaryngeal intubation, tracheostomy exibits many advantages:[2-4]

- Improvement of patients' comfort, while being better tolerated
- Reduction of patients' analgosedation needs
- Improvement of communication
- Possibility of swallowing
- Reduction of accidental endotracheal tube dislocations
- Better airway security and reduction of risks of airway loss in cases of difficult intubation
- No necessity of anesthesia/sedation for airway exchange maneuvers
- Improvement and facilitation of oropharyngeal nursing
- Reduction of airway obstruction
- Reduction of sinusitis incidence
- Possible benefit in terms of respiratory tract infection reduction.

During 1970's, the observation of a large number of stenotic tracheal complications shifted the use

of tracheostomy towards the use of prolonged translaryngeal intubation, but since the early 90's elective tracheostomy came back to be a common practice in ICUs, even because of percutaneous techniques widespread diffusion.

Percutaneous technique was firstly described 20 years ago by the thoracic surgeon Pasquale Ciaglia, who used a multiple dilators technique, similar to percutaneous nephrostomy technique, for progressive soft tissue dilation.[5] The aim for research and development of a new tracheostomy technique was to avoid the severe complications of surgical tracheostomy, described up to middle 80's and later,[6] and to reduce the incidence of minor complications such as non-esthetic scar and stomal infections, which characterized surgical technique in the following years.[7] Percutaneous technique allowed bedside procedure in critical and difficult to move patients and required less time and few operators, even without specific surgical skills, to be performed, thus resulting in a more effective and cost saving procedure.

For these reasons percutaneous dilational tracheostomy is now a days the most used technique to perform tracheostomy in ICU patients.[8]

Several techniques have been introduced and tested during the last 20 years, but only a few of them resulted effective. The majority of percutaneous approaches require a transcervical or anterograde approach using a guidewire technique as introduced by Seldinger more than 50 years ago for vascular cannulation; the only techniques using a different approach are represented by percutaneous procedures developed before Ciaglia technique and by translaryngeal technique described by Fantoni,[9] in which a dedicated cannula premounted on a traction wire is used instead of dilators on guidewire technique to allow an inner to outer traction.

Indeed many of the reasons justifying introduction of percutaneous technique might not be considered furtherly actual: as an example, rapidity of the procedure has lost its importance if considering percutaneous tracheostomy as an elective procedure which should be performed with the maximum safety and under continuous endoscopic control.

In case of emergency, a simpler cricothyroid membrane access should be preferable, and if considered in terms of costs-benefits, the declared lower cost of percutaneous techniques has played in Italy a minor role if compared with other countries.[10]

If comparing the standard surgical and the different percutaneous techniques, the results are often conflicting, of difficult interpretation and often unattendable for several reasons:[11]

- Lack of univocal definitions for both procedural standards and complications; as an example periprocedural bleeding has been both quantitatively or semi quantitatively defined in the most different terms
- Lack of standard criteria for timing, patient enrollment (including anatomical landmarks detection) or for procedural phases; as an example dilation performed with or without preliminary dissection, with or without continuous endoscopic control or with more or less defined and individual variations of the basic technique

- Difference and lack of homogeneity of underlying pathologies of patients receiving tracheostomy
- Predefined patient selection
- Statistical and methodological differences between studies
- Lack or great variety of follow-up standards and criteria.

Between the most commonly used percutaneous techniques, the rotational procedure is a recently introduced single dilator technique showing growing success and diffusion. Designed in Italy in 2001[12,13] it was realized and distributed by Ruesch (now Teleflex Medical), Kernen, Germany, and introduced in the European market in 2002 with the trademark PercuTwist™; it is based on an original and radically different dilational concept, as the opportune pathway between skin and trachea is established thanking to a progressive controlled dilation obtained with a dedicated screw dilator of variable caliber (Fig. 8.1), under continuous endoscopic control.

Procedure Description

The tracheotomy should be performed in general anesthesia by intravenous technique in 100% oxygen. The procedure should not be performed

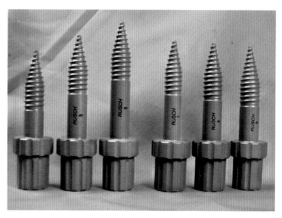

Fig. 8.1: Screw single dilators of different size and length. Commercial versions are sizes 7, 8 and 9 with a standard length (right side)

without continuous endoscopic control, and this suggestion should be adopted for all percutaneous techniques, even if also recent papers seem to ignore this prudent safety rule.[14,15]

Continuous endoscopy allows:

a. Identification of possible laryngeal or tracheal lesions due to prolonged intubation
b. Transillumination of cervical region and identification of anterior blood vessels[16]
c. Correct needle placement at the beginning of the procedure
d. Protection against posterior wall lesions or false routes[17]
e. Visual control of cannula insertion
f. Tracheal exploration by entering the cannula at the end of procedure for position confirmation
g. Limitation or immediate identification of tracheal rings lesions.

Airway control during the procedure can be secured with different strategies:

a. Endotracheal tube removal and, after careful pharyngeal aspiration, positioning of LMA classic (Authors' preferred solution) or any other extraglottic device which allows fiberscope passage
b. Partial retraction of endotracheal tube up to the direct vision of the cuff in the laryngeal inlet, if necessary granting airway control maintenance via a tube-exchanger
c. Endotracheal tube removal under direct laryngoscopy and replacement with a larger one, the tube's tip in the laryngeal inlet and the tube's cuff in hypopharynx.

Head position can be indifferent, without any need of hyperextension or use of a pillow below the patient's shoulders; both these conditions, together with anterior neck pressure during tracheostomy might in fact represent causes of undesired intracranial pressure rising. In the original technique head is just fixed in the neutral position using a dedicated wrap passing by the chin (Fig. 8.2). Sterile field preparation should be

extremely careful, as the tight adhesion between neck tissues and tracheostomy cannula observed in all percutaneous techniques with small skin incision would not allow opportune drainage in case of wound infection (more frequent with the standard surgical technique rather than with percutaneous techniques.[14] Local anesthesia plus adrenaline infiltration is not routinely used.

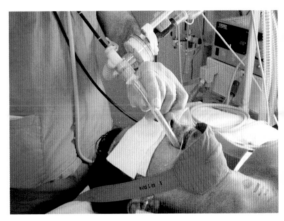

Fig. 8.2 : Chin fixation

Needle insertion should be performed between cricoid cartilage and the third tracheal ring with a dedicated 14 G cannula-over-the-needle provided in the commercial kit. The choice for the cricoid cartilage – first ring interspace might be possible in case of short term translaryngeal intubation before tracheostomy and in absence of endoscopic evidence of cricoid cartilage sufferance; this site of puncture might allow avoidance of head hyperextension in case of "short" or "difficult" neck and the consequent institution of a long and non rectilinear skin-tracheal route, responsible for difficult cannula exchange and possible later adherences between the trachea and anterior neck tissues resulting in swallowing interference.

The needle should always be inserted perpendicularly to the skin, in a previously endoscopically identified site, always on the midline and mandatorily in the interanular space.

Guidewire insertion is possible once the access cannula is in position, similarly to other percutaneous techniques. The length and diameter characteristics of *Percutwist*™ guidewire make it different and less prone to kinking if compared with other commercial sets. Guidewire regular progression should be fiberoptically controlled.

The next step is a small *skin incision*, either horizontal or vertical (Authors' preference), no more than 6-10 mm wide according to the tracheostomic cannula diameter. There is no need to perform skin incisions wider than the cannula outer diameter, which might only result in the loss of the tight adhesion between the cannula itself and soft tissues. The choice between horizontal or vertical incision is only determined by the evidence of blood vessels previously identified by transillumination (Fig. 8.3) and by the choice of eventual preliminary ligation. Long time outcomes of either horizontal or vertical skin incisions are equally favorable.[16]

Dilation is performed by progressive clockwise rotation of the PercuTwist™ screw, gradually deepening in soft tissues and leaving it free to follow the guidewire direction. The PercuTwist™ screw is commercially available for 7, 8, 9 mm ID cannulas insertion (respectively corresponding to an outer screw diameter of 11.6–13.0 and 14.3 mm),

and is coated with an hydrophilic film with lubricating properties activated once the conic part of the screw itself is immersed in water for no more than 15-20 seconds. During the first 2 or 3 turns of the screw, a moderate pressure might be applied, in order to allow the screw to grasp tissues; during the following progression no pressure application is needed. Conversely, the rotation should be performed while applying an upwards lift with 2nd and 3rd finger of the non-dominating hand opened as a "V" below the screw handle, as showed in Fig. 8.4. This movement allows an outer directed traction on pretracheal tissues, resulting in the anterior tracheal wall staying far from the posterior tracheal wall with a reduced risk of posterior wall lesions and the possibility of a controlled dilation.

Every complete screw turn corresponds to 2.5 mm advancement; normally the screw's tip appears in the tracheal lumen in a mean time of 40 seconds; this passage might be felt by skilled hands as a different sensation of resistance, but the definitive confirmation must be obtained fiberoptically. The dilator's correct progression and position and guidewire integrity should be regularly checked during advancement; this may be obtained performing a repeated "to and from" guidewire's movement through the dilator in position, which

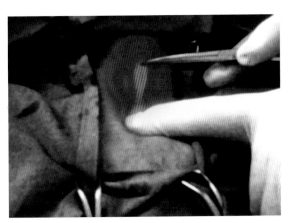

Fig. 8.3: Blood vessels evidenced by transillumination

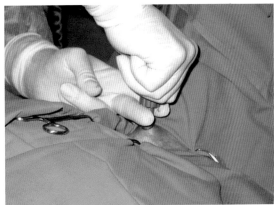

Fig. 8.4: Two fingers dilator lift during rotation

must be perceived as smooth and obstacle-free. Once the screw's tip appears in the trachea, the dilator's progression might be continued while gently bending the screw itself towards the patient's chin always under fiberoptic control, even if the operator's sensation should always be to let the screw naturally follow the guidewire. Rotation is stopped as soon as the whole conic part of the screw (corresponding to 6-7 screw lines to be counted fiberoptically) is visible into the tracheal lumen (Fig. 8.5); the screw is then counter-clockwise rotated without any traction until its complete removal.

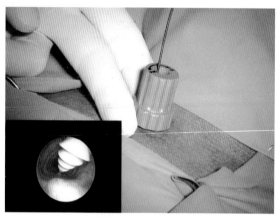

Fig. 8.5: The whole conic part into the tracheal lumen

The *tracheostomy cannula insertion* is performed over an introducer, whose characteristics (shape, stiffness, length, sliding surface) might influence both the need for pushing to introduce the cannula and the risk for distal tracheal lesions. The actual commercial kit provides a semi-rigid round-tipped introducer with a stop-ring in the proximal part aimed to limit the introducer's protrusion over the cannula itself. The introducer and cannula should be preassembled and lubricated; the cannula's cuff inflated, checked, deflated and retired "parachute-like" towards the proximal part (Fig. 8.6) before starting the procedure, so that after screw removal the cannula-introducer is ready

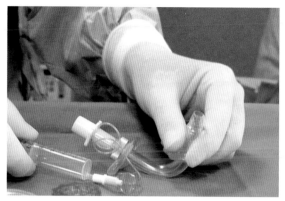

Fig. 8.6: "Parachute-like" cuff retraction

to be railroaded on the guidewire. In order to make insertion easier, a two hand push might be adopted, with one hand on the introducer and the other on the cannula, just following the curved shape of the route. As an exclusive characteristic of this technique, the tracheal stoma just after the screw removal remains dilated, granting the need of a lower pressure push to insert the tracheostomy cannula if compared with other techniques.

After fiberoptic control of the trachea and flange position adjustment (the commercial kit provides both a fixed and an adjustable-flange tracheostomy cannula) the *cannula is fixed* accordingly to various techniques, including, though rarely, a two stitches skin suture whenever the neck morphology prevents the use of traditional dedicated wraps. Medication necessity is minimal, and could be avoided after the first 24 hours.

The *cannula exchange* procedure, except for technical defects, is not routinely made, but generally it should be advisable to wait several days as a safe time lag necessary to stabilize the stomal route enough to left the stoma temporarily patent despite the absence of the cannula. It is important to remark that in all procedures with a tight adhesion between cannula and tissues, such as many percutaneous techniques, at least 5-7 days, or even more, are necessary to stabilize the stomal route.

The advantage of such adhesion is the low infection rate and the low incidence of bleeding, the most important disadvantage being the risk of airway loss in case of accidental decannulation in non-ICU setting. For such reasons percutaneous tracheostomy should be reserved to patients expected to stay in ICU for at least one week.

While the surgical technique grants the stoma patency thanking to stitches at the sides of the stoma or the suture to the skin of a cartilaginous window, thus allowing a relatively easy cannula reinsertion, the same maneuver in case of percutaneous tracheostomy might be more difficult, thus requiring a *protected procedure*, such as using a small size uncuffed endotracheal tube, a suction catheter, a rectal probe, a dedicated cannula-exchanger or a fiberscope-Aintree[TM] (Cook) to remove the old and to railroad the new cannula in the correct position (with preference to any device which might allow periprocedural oxygenation). In absence of specific skills or in risky situations (night time, acute oxygen desaturation, etc.) a safe choice could to perform traditional translaryngeal intubation and delay reinsertion of cannula until airway is secured.

Difficulties in cannula exchange procedures might be even longer lasting in chronically ill domiciliated patients, without any possibility of prompt medical intervention. For these reasons, standard surgical tracheostomy remains an advisable procedure in this kind of patients, or in extremely obese patients, in smaller children and generally in all anatomically difficult situations, whenever dedicated skills and experience are missing.

Programmed decannulation for rotational technique is similar to the one followed for the surgical technique; generally it must be persuaded gradually, even if, differently from the surgical approach, no stitches or tapes are necessary to approach wound edges, because of the marked tendency to spontaneous closure.

Considerations

After a 4 years experience, the rotational procedure proved to be a simple and easy to learn technique; after the preliminary cases reported in 2002,[13] the results of a 3 years period (2002-2005) have been recently published.[16] While being an easy to learn and easy to perform procedure, similarly to other percutaneous tracheostomies, this technique requires a minimum surgical knowledge and some experience and dexterity.

A retrospective analysis on 348 PercuTwist[TM] tracheostomies showed the complete absence of major complications and less than 10% minor complications: 1.1% procedure revision because of bleeding, 1.4% of guidewire kinking (up to 2003, that is with the old model "green" guidewire, since then changed with the non kinking "blue" one) and 5.4 % tracheal ring rupture. An affordable difficulty in rotation was recorded in 8.04% of cases and in 1.72% a difficulty in cannula insertion was reported.

Especially immediately after its introduction, different objections were raised to this new technique:

- Yet in the preliminary report[13] a certain *rotation difficulty* and the skin rotation together with the screw dilator were reported. This finding was more common in young black patients with relatively inelastic skin (Fig. 8.7) or in elderly patients with overabundant skin. While the skin rotation has a low clinical relevance, the problem of *rotational resistance*, initially responsible of technique withdrawal,[18-20] was completely solved in 2004 after the introduction of a diameter magnifying ring (Fig. 8.8) to be mounted on the screw handle. Such a ring, enlarging the handle diameter from 25 to 35 mm, allows to overcome even high resistances despite the same strength appliance.
- A significant and relatively frequent difficulty in *cannula insertion* during the final phases of the procedure has also been described; in two cases[18] the difficulty was so high to become

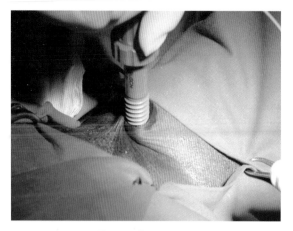

Fig. 8.7: Skin rotation

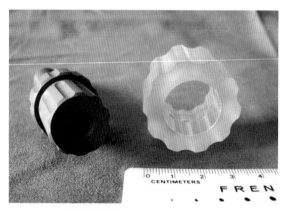

Fig. 8.8: Diameter magnifying ring

responsible of guidewire kinking and major complications (cardiac arrest and tracheo-oesophageal fistula). These complications are due to limited experience with the technique and, as reported by the same authors, to the high pressures exerted by the operator on the dilator screw until its tip reached the tracheal lumen. Since 2004 the guidewire was radically redesigned, making it much more resistant to kinking, and the simple tip of checking its free "to and from" movement during rotation, make unnecessary any downwards pressure or strength application if not for the first screw

turn in the subcutaneous tissues.[21] Conversely, the previously reported problem might depend on incomplete dilational procedure before attempting cannula insertion; more rarely (1.72% in our experience[16] depended on excessive introducer flexibility, observed during the intermediate productive phase of the new commercial kit.

- While this technique has been recognized the advantage of avoiding any tracheal compression during dilational phase, some reports indicated *posterior tracheal wall lesions*, anyway.[18,22] Excluding all lesions depending on unnecessary downwards pressure application during rotation, a careful analysis of the above mentioned reports allows a relative exclusion of rotational dilation procedure between the possible lesion dynamics,[16] very similarly due to the cannula insertion procedure, which represents a common risk for all percutaneous anterograde techniques. The absence of major complications, including false posterior routes, when considering wide sampled studies[16,20,21,23] rather than anecdotal reports, represents an important safety warranty for this technique.

- A minor complication commonly observed in all percutaneous tracheostomy techniques is represented by *cartilaginous structure lesions*, occurring with an incidence ranging from 2 to 8.9% with an isolated (and difficult to understand) 36% reported for BlueRhino™ (Cook) technique.[18] According to literature, both isolated cases[24-26] or different percentages in larger studies have been reported for the PercuTwist™ technique: 2% over 100 cases;[27] slightly more than 5% over 348 cases;[16] 12% over 54 cases;[23] 10% over 35 cases;[28] 2% in the 90 cases reported by Sengupta and coworkers;[21] 2.7% in Bewsher and coworkers[29] and 0% in a recent paper comparing PercuTwist, Griggs and Ciaglia's techniques.[30] This complication is not considered as clinically relevant for percutaneous techniques[7,31,32] even if some authors report cases of possible tracheomalacic evolution[33] or distal fragments migration.[34]

- Despite using different percutaneous techniques (Fantoni, Griggs, Ciaglia and Blue Rhino™) the larger incidence of periprocedural complications has been described[35] for the *largely obese patient* if compared to normal subjects, despite some differences between Authors.[36] A multicentric trial on PercuTwist™ technique[20] showed that, whenever the skin-trachea distance exceeded 4.5 cm, some operators changed technique or implemented other techniques. Even if these cases are actually rare in Italy, as the largely obese population seems to be growing, a new screw with an additional 1 cm length was studied and probably available in the future (Fig. 8.1).

- The rotational technique, similar to few others percutaneous techniques[32,36] might be performed closely to recent surgical wounds, or in recent traumatic brain injury, as it does not require head hyperextension or neck pressure, thus resulting in lack of periprocedural intracranial pressure increase.[37] In a recent study, Imperiale et al have used Percutwist tracheostomy technique in 65 consecutive critically ill patients admitted to the neurosurgical ICU. They observed that the brain-injured patients with stable ICP (<20 mm Hg) did not have clinically significantly increase in ICP or $PaCO_2$ and was not associated with neurological deterioration.[38]

CONCLUSION

Percutaneous techniques, and particularly the five techniques using a single dilator approach (Griggs, Ciaglia, Fantoni,[9] Frova[12,13] and the most recent Ambesh[39,40]) progressively took the place of standard surgical technique in ICU patients. Despite such a diffusion, even for the apparently easiest techniques such as the above described, operators experience and ability to convert at any moment a percutaneous in surgical tracheostomy remain mandatory. Only with this approach we might have certainty not only to abolish major complications thanking to technique's safety but also to limit as much as possible the incidence of minor complications, which remain constantly operator-dependent.

Thus percutaneous dilational techniques can not be simply considered as an alternative to surgical technique because of ward's local habits, but most importantly as a preferential and elective choice for all ICU intubated patients with the exception of small children and sometimes of chronically ventilator dependent respiratory patients. The rationale for rotational percutaneous tracheostomy remain the procedure simplicity, the low rate of both infections and non-esthetic scars, the need for minimal nursing and the possibility to anticipate it in comparison with past habits even in recent traumatic brain injury patients.

REFERENCES

1. Pierson DJ. Tracheostomy from A to Z. Historical context and current challenges. Respir Care 2005;50: 473-5.
2. El-Naggar M, Sadagopan S, Levine H, et al. Factors influencing choice between tracheostomy and prolonged translaryngeal intubation in acute respiratory failure: A prospective study. Anesth Analg 1976;55:195-201.
3. Stauffer JL, Olson DE, Petty TL. Complications and consequences of endotracheal intubation and tracheotomy. Am J Med 1981;70:65-76.
4. Dunham CM, La Monica C. Prolonged tracheal intubation in the trauma patient. J Trauma 1984;24: 120-4.
5. Ciaglia P, Firshing R, Syniec C. Elective percutaneous dilatational tracheostomy: A new simple bedside procedure; preliminary report. Chest 1985;87:715-9.
6. Goldenberg D, Gov Ari E, Goiz A, et al. Tracheotomy complications: a retrospective study of 1130 cases. Arch Otolaryngol Head Neck Surg 2000;123:495-500.
7. Gysin C, Dulguerov P, Guyot JP, et al. Percutaneous versus surgical tracheostomy. A double-blind randomized trial. Annals of Surgery 1999;230:708-14.

8. GIVITI. Progetto Margherita 2004; www.marionegri.it

9. Fantoni A, Ripamonti D. Tracheostomia translaringea: Metodo non chirurgico. Intensive Care Medicine 1997;3:193-8.

10. Levin R, Trivikram L. Cost/benefit analysis of open tracheotomy, in the OR and at the bedside, with percutaneous tracheotomy. Laryngoscope 2001; 111:1169-73.

11. Gullo A, Sorbello M, Frova G. Percutaneous versus surgical tracheostomy: An unfinished symphony. Critical Care Medicine 2007;35:682-3.

12. Frova G. Improvements in percutaneous tracheostomy: The single-step rotational dilation. 16th Apice. Gullo A (Ed), Springer Verlag, Milano 2002:305-13.

13. Frova G, Quintel M. A new simple method for percutaneous tracheostomy: Controlled rotating dilation. Intensive Care Med 2002;28:299-303.

14. Silvester W, Goldsmith D, Uchino S, et al. Percutaneous versus surgical tracheostomy: A randomized controlled study with long-term follow-up. Crit Care Med 2006; 34:2145-52.

15. Paran H, Butnaru G, Hass I, et al. Evaluation of a modified percutaneous tracheostomy technique without bronchoscopic guidance. Chest 2004;126:868-71.

16. Frova G, Galbiati P, Barozzi O, et al. Percutaneous rotational tracheostomy (Percutwist): analysis of 348 consecutive procedures. Journal Anaesthesie Intensivbehandlung 2006;3:19-22.

17. Marelli D, Paul A, Manolidis S, et al. Endoscopic guided percutaneous tracheostomy: Early results of a consecutive trial. J Trauma 1990;30:433-5.

18. Byhahn C, Westphal K, Meininger D, et al. Single-dilator percutaneous tracheostomy. A comparison of PercuTwist and Ciaglia Blue Rhino techniques. Intensive Care Medicine 2002;28:1262-6.

19. Fikkers BG, Venwiel JM, Tillmans RJ. Percutaneous tracheostomy with the Percutwist technique not so easy. Anaesthesia 2002;57:935-6.

20. Frova G, Terenghi P, Barozzi O, et al. PercuTwist: 2 years of clinical experience. Minerva Anestesiologica 2003;52:95-9.

21. Sengupta N, Ang KL, Prakash, et al. Twenty months' use of a new percutaneous tracheostomy set using controlled rotating dilation. Anesth Analg 2004;99:188-92.

22. Thant M, Samuel T. Posterior tracheal wall tear with Percutwist. Anaesthesia 2002;57:507-8.

23. Grundling M, Kuhn SO, Nees J, et al. PercuTwist-Dilatation tracheotomie. Prospektive evaluation an 54 konsecutiven patienten. Anaesthesist 2004;53:434-40.

24. Byhahn C, Wilke HJ, Halbig S, et al. Percutaneous tracheostomy: Ciaglia Blue Rhino vs the basic Ciaglia technique of percutaneous dilational tracheostomy. Anesth Analg 2000;91:882-6.

25. Roberts RG, Morgan P, Findlay GP. Percutaneous dilatational tracheostomy and tracheal ring rupture. Anaesthesia 2002;57:933.

26. Edwards SM, Williams JC. Tracheal cartilage fracture with the blue Rhino Ciaglia percutaneous tracheostomy system. Eur J Anaesth 2001;18:487.

27. Quintel M, Frova G. Anaesthesia 2002,57:933.

28. Kinner JA, Higgins DJ. Tracheal ring fracture and herniation with PercuTwist percutaneous dilator. Thorac Cardiovasc Surg 2000;120:329-34.

29. Bewsher MS, Adams AM, Clarke CWM, et al. Evaluation of a new percutaneous dilatational tracheostomy set. Anaesthesia 2000; 56:859-64.

30. Yurtseven N, Aydemir B, Karaca P, et al. Percutwist: A new alternative to Griggs and Ciaglia's techniques. Eur J Anaesth 2007;8:1-6.

31. Hazard P, Jones C, Benitone J. Comparative clinical trial of standard operative tracheostomy with percutaneous tracheostomy. Crit Care Med 1991; 19:1018-24.

32. Byhahn C, Rinne T, Halbig S, et al. Early percutaneous tracheostomy after median sternotomy. J Thorac Cardiovasc Surg 2000;120:329-34.

33. Ho EC, Kapila A, Colquhoun-Flannery W. Tracheal ring fracture and early tracheomalacia following percutaneous dilatational tracheostomy. BMC Ear, Nose and Throat Disorders 2005;5:634) Scherrer E, Tual L, Dhonneur G. Tracheal Ring fracture during a PercuTwist tracheostomy procedure. Anesth Analg 2004;98:1451-3.

34. Byhahn C, Lischke V, Meininger D, et al. Peri operative complications during percutaneous tracheostomy in obese patients. Anaesthesia 2005;60:12-5.

35. Mansharamani NG, Koziel H, Garland R, et al. Safety of bedside percutaneous dilatational tracheostomy in obese patients in the ICU. Chest 2000;117:1426-9.

36. Patel NC, Deane J, Scawn N. Reduction in tracheostomy-associated risk of mediastinitis by routine use of percutaneous tracheostomy. Ann Thorac Surg 2002;73:2033(letter).

37. De Blasiis N, Imperiale C, Baisi F, et al. New technique for percutaneous tracheostomy in neurosurgical patients: preliminary cases. The Journal of ASA 2003; A-446.

38. Imperiale C, Magni G, Favaro R, Rosa G. Intracranial monitoring during percutaneous tracheostomy "Percutwist" in critically ill neurosurgery patients. Anesth Analg 2009;108:588-92.

39. Ambesh SP. A new percutaneous tracheostomy kit "Ambesh T-Dagger". Journal Anaesthesie Intensivbehandlung 2006;3:22-5.

40. Ambesh SP, Tripathi M, Pandey CK, Pant KC, Singh PK. Clinical evaluation of the "T-Dagger": A new bedside percutaneous dilational tracheostomy device. Anaesthesia 2005;60:708-11.

Fantoni's Translaryngeal Tracheostomy Technique

Donata Ripamonti

INTRODUCTION

Translaryngeal tracheostomy (TLT) is a non-derivative technique whose main feature is the passage of a dilator from the inside of the trachea to the outside of the neck (Fig. 9.1), while all others follow an exactly opposite direction and thus it has been defined as Outside-Inside Tracheostomy (OIT). It is therefore a true innovation rather than a modification or evolution of existing techniques.

The TLT was presented at first by Fantoni in 1993 [1], in a version very different from the final version proposed in 1997.[2] The first TLT method was based on a progressive and fractional dilation and was performed by means of a home-made tool, named familiarly "rosary", formed by a series of metallic cones, 1 to 2.5 cm long and with an increasing diameter from 3 to 15 mm, inserted in a metallic wire at a distance of 20 cm, from one to the other. An armoured and flexible cannula was joined to the final cone and was dragged by it from the inside of the trachea to the outside the neck (Fig. 9.2).

The entire maneuvre was performed in apnea, but there was in every moment the possibility to intubate and ventilate the patient after the passage of each cones, thanks to the distance between them.

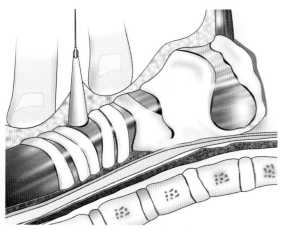

Fig. 9.1: Translaryngeal tracheostomy

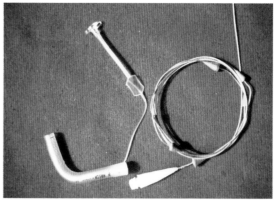

Fig. 9.2: The rosary

In a second time, the multiple cones were replaced by a unique dilator, joined to a cannula. This device (Fig. 9.3) was first used in a child in which, the TLT was performed not in apnea, but with manual respiratory assistance by means of a small ventilation catheter.

In a third time, a tool for the adult was performed, with a single cone joined to the armoured and flexible cannula (Fig. 9.4), and in this way the first "cone-cannula" was conceived, the instrument that characterized the translaryngeal tracheostomy. Also in adult patients, the TLT was performed not in apnea, but with mechanical or manual respiratory assistance by means of a small ventilation catheter.

Subsequently the necessary material for TLT was supplied in a kit, now supplied by Covidien Healthcare SPA (Fig. 9.5).

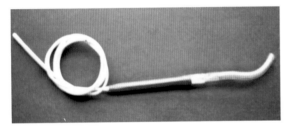

Fig. 9.3: The unique dilator

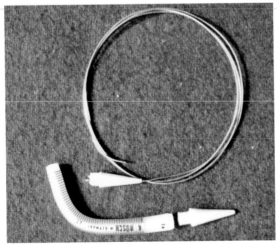

Fig. 9.4: The first home made "cone-cannula"

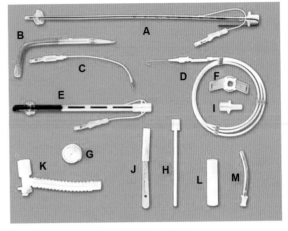

Fig. 9.5: The TLT kit

A : Cuffed ventilation catheter
B : Cone-cannula
C : Cuff inflation line
D : J wire
E : Rigid tracheoscope (RTS)
F : Cannula adapter
G : Fixation tape
H : Obturator
I : Cannula connector
J : Lancet
K : Catheter mount
L : Pull handle
M : Curved needle

The three principal instruments are the cuffed ventilation catheter, the rigid tracheoscope (RTS) and the cone-cannula, the original instrument of the TLT kit (Fig. 9.6).

The cuffed cannula is of the armoured, very flexible type, moulded together with the cone of soft plastic material which ends with a hollow metallic point (Fig. 9.7).

The short cuff is located at the end of the cannula to facilitate tracheal insertion of the cannula itself. The cannula is available in the sizes 5.5, 6.5, 7.5, 8.5, 9.5 mm ID. We use 7.5–8.5 mm ID for adults, 5.5–6.5 mm ID for younger people. There is also a kit with a straight cannula.

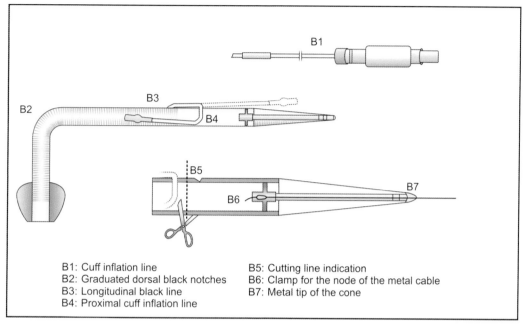

B1: Cuff inflation line
B2: Graduated dorsal black notches
B3: Longitudinal black line
B4: Proximal cuff inflation line

B5: Cutting line indication
B6: Clamp for the node of the metal cable
B7: Metal tip of the cone

Fig. 9.6: The cone-cannula

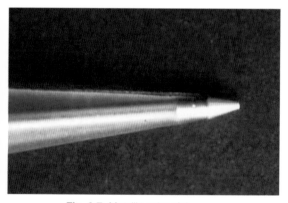

Fig. 9.7: Metallic point of the cone

The cuffed ventilation catheter is a small tube, with a high volume low pressure cuff so as to create a perfect seal in the circuit and therefore high peak inspiratory pressure (PIP) or positive end expiratory pressure (PEEP) may be maintained, if required. The ventilation catheter is supplied in three sizes: 3, 4 and 5 mm ID accordingly to the size of the cannula.

The rigid tracheoscope is made in transparent plastic with a black tip so as to increase contrast with tracheal mucosa, making positioning extremely precise. It is fitted with a cuff, slightly back from the tip so as to avoid perforation by the needle. A longitudinal black line indicates the shortest edge of the flute-shaped tip and thus the orientation of the oblique opening of the instrument (Fig. 9.8).

The needle is also a particular device, curved so as to permit its retrograde insertion that characterises the TLT. Another feature of this needle is the rounded, virtually blunt tip that essentially helps to separate the highly vascularised tissues of the neck, with the advantage of significantly reducing the risk of hemorrhage.

Preferred Technique

In the first official presentation of the translaryngeal tracheostomy supported by a significant series of patients [2] several possible modalities of performing the procedure were illustrated with a first,

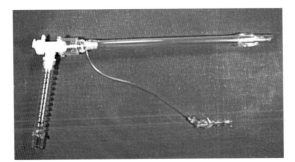

Fig. 9.8: The rigid tracheoscope (RTS)

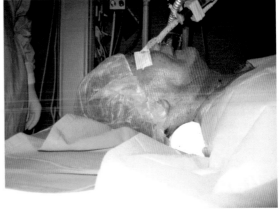

Fig. 9.9: TLT head position

provisional evaluation of each one of them. Subsequently, it was realized that only one of these modalities proved entirely suitable to the principle which prompted Fantoni to invent a new technique: the highest intrinsic, non operator-dependent safety, the least local trauma and full control of the maneuvres. Therefore, we have adopted this modality as the exclusive procedure to perform TLT, and defined it as the basic technique.

An original subdivision in phases, suitable for all kinds of percutaneous methods,[3] will be adopted to accomplish a detailed description, step by step, of the technique (Table 9.1).

Table 9.1: Subdivision into phases of percutaneous tracheostomy		
Phase 1	Phase 2	Phase 3
needle insertion	dilation	Cannula placement

Phase 1: Needle Insertion

The team of operators is formed by two anesthesiologists (like intensivists are in our country) and a nurse. The patient is subjected to general intravenous anesthesia, neuromuscular blockade, 100% oxygen ventilation and standard cardiorespiratory monitoring. A pillow, if necessary, is placed under the head to line up the oral, laryngeal and tracheal axis. The neck is not hyperextended (Fig. 9.9).

After the removal of the endotracheal tube (ETT) and a thorough assessment of the laryngeal and tracheal condition, the RTS is inserted into the trachea. A slight turning on the left of the head and a lateral retromolar entry (Fig. 9.10) make the maneuvre easier.

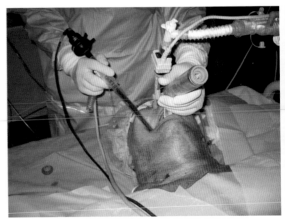

Fig. 9.10: Retromolar entry

A 0° telescope allows advancing the tip of the RTS, with extreme precision, as far as the selected interannular space of trachea. With a leverage, the end of the instrument is pushed upward giving the possibility to be palpated from the outside (Fig. 9.11).

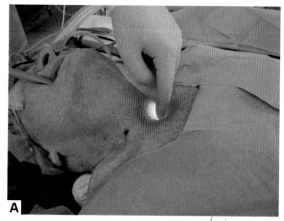

A

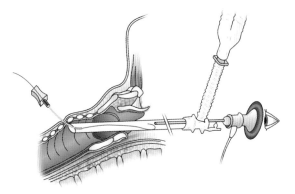

Fig. 9.12: Needle and wire insertion and advancement inside the RTS

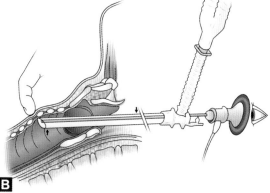

B

Fig. 9.11: The leverage of RTS enhances the transillumination and ensures palpation of the end of RTS from the outside

The curved needle is then inserted into the bulging area. As the point of the needle appears inside, the tracheoscope is turned in a way that the oval opening is faced upwards to facilitate the direct advancement of the needle, 2-3 cm inside its lumen but especially to protect the posterior wall of the trachea. The wire is made to run inside the RTS and is recovered at the tube connector (Fig. 9.12).

The needle is then removed; the RTS is removed too and replaced by a small ventilation catheter (Fig. 9.13).

The J-segment of the wire is cut away and the cone is threaded with the wire that is then extracted from the lateral slot of the cannula. A length of silk safety thread is joined to the wire and the knot is

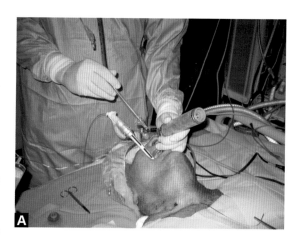

A

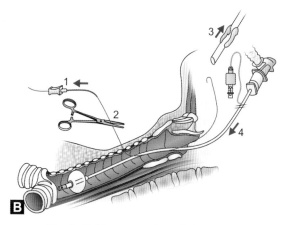

B

Fig. 9.13: Placement of ventilation catheter

pulled inside the cannula. This "safety thread" enables the repetition of the full procedure in the event of early accidental decannulation (Fig. 9.14).

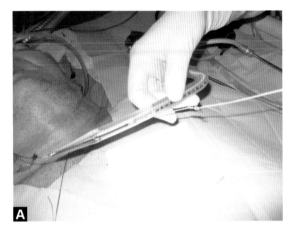

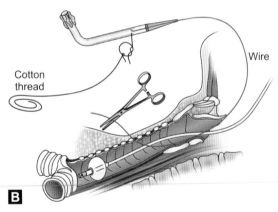

Fig. 9.14: Wire and safety thread connection to the cone-cannula

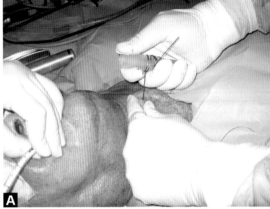

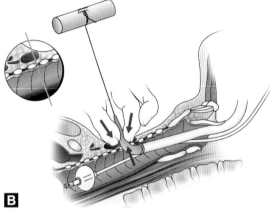

Fig. 9.15A and B: Cone-cannula extraction

Phase 2: Stage of Dilation

By pulling on the end of the wire going out of the neck, by means of a specific instrument supplied in the kit, the cone-cannula is dragged through the larynx and neck wall. The pressure of the fingers should be only enough to prevent an upwards displacement of the tissue layers (Fig. 9.15).

As the metal tip of the cone emerges, 1 to 2 mm long incisions on the constricting tissue ring are made to reduce resistance, more to facilitate

the rotation of the cannula, in the following phase, rather than the extraction of the cone. The extraction of the cone-cannula is continued until one half of the length of the cannula is extracted (Fig. 9.16).

Phase 3: Cannula Placement

After separating the cone from the cannula (Fig. 9.17), a 0° telescope is inserted into the cannula as far as the curving of the cannula permits (Fig. 9.18).

By making the cannula slide along the telescope, the extraction is gradually resumed (Fig. 9.19).

When the posterior wall appears at the bottom (Fig. 9.20), it means the cannula is fully straightened and can be rotated and advanced downwards, always under direct endoscopic view (Fig. 9.21).

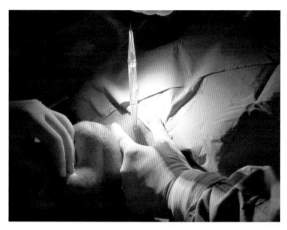

Fig. 9.16: One half of the cannula is extracted

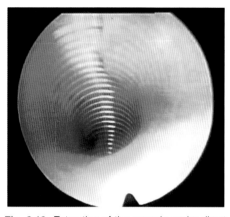

Fig. 9.19: Extraction of the cannula under direct endoscopic control

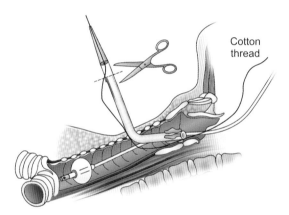

Cotton thread

Fig. 9.17: Cone-cannula separation

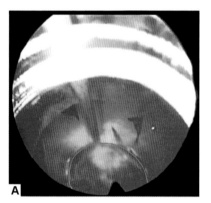

Fig. 9.20: Posterior tracheal wall

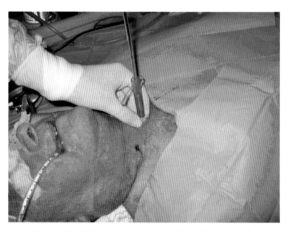

Fig. 9.18: 0° telescope inserted into the cannula

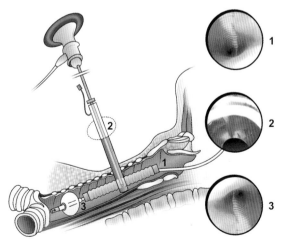

Fig. 9.21: Extraction (1), straightening (2) rotation and final positioning (3) of the cannula

The identification of the tracheal lumen allows one to remove the catheter and to start the ventilation through the tracheal cannula.

Ventilation

The ventilation is maintained for the whole length of the procedure, by means of RTS in phase 1 and with the ventilation catheter in Phases 2 and 3. The correct placement into the inferior half of the trachea of the ventilation catheter and the fitness of the respiratory support may be checked by the simple lung auscultation and thorax movements. The respirator setting should be obviously adapted, in Phases 2 and 3, to the higher resistances by lowering the frequency and raising the inspiratory pressure to maintain an adequate tidal volume and a plateau pressure ≤ 35 cm H_2O. The previous PEEP is maintained unchanged.

The continuity of ventilation and the availability of a closed respiratory circuit enable one to carry out the TLT even in patients with the most severe acute lung injury, demanding high PIP and PEEP.

Other Possible Variations of the Technique

Phase 1: The insertion of the needle, obviously directed cranially, can also be made with the use of a flexible fiberscope (FFB), with the same scheme used for all other outside/inside percutaneous techniques (OITs). The wire is advanced cranially aside the endotracheal tube, after deflating the cuff, and then recovered with forceps in the oral cavity (Fig. 9.22). After connecting the wire to the cone-cannula the ETT is replaced by the ventilation catheter.

Some users prefer to steer the wire directly into the lumen of the ETT and recover its end at the tube connector. In this case the ETT should be replaced by the ventilation catheter before making the wire–cone connection (Fig. 9.23).

These variations are probably the most widespread modality to implement the needle

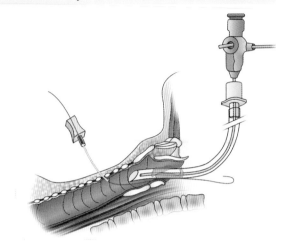

Fig. 9.22: Advancement of the wire cranially aside the endotracheal tube after deflating the cuff

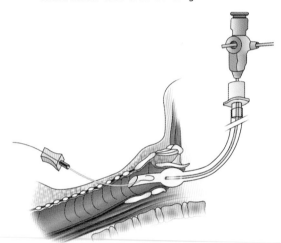

Fig. 9.23: Advancement of the wire directly into the lumen of the endotracheal tube

introduction among the TLT users. The lack of familiarity with optical rigid instruments is the principal factor of the FFB choice.

Phase 2: There are no variations

Phase 3: The straightening and rotation maneuvre can be performed by making the cannula slip along the obturator of the kit (Fig. 9.24). In this case, the checking of the internal shift of the cannula, to be considered mandatory, is made with an optical instrument from the oral cavity (Figs 9.25 and 9.26).

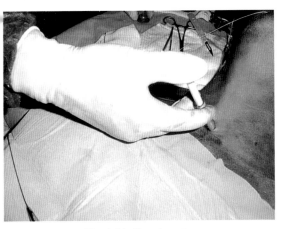

Fig. 9.24: The obturator

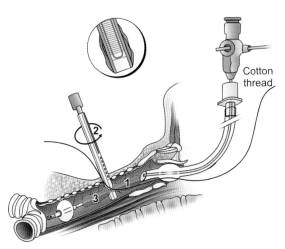

Cotton thread

Fig. 9.25: Checking with optical lens

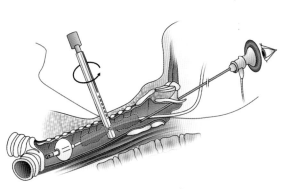

Fig. 9.26: Checking with fibrescope

Advantages of TLT Method

Phase 1: The rigid tracheoscope, employed in the great majority of cases, provides many benefits. Its levering enhances the transillumination (Fig. 9.11) by reducing the thickness of the pretracheal tissue. With the leverage of the instrument, the trachea is pulled cranially, the palpation of the edge of the distal end of the RTS, positioned at the chosen level, precisely selected from the inside, exempts the operator from finding the neck landmarks.

The RTS immobilizes the trachea, blocks its lateral and downward shifting, so that the centring of the needle becomes precise and rapid. The tracheal walls are kept far from each other. The upwards turning of the distal opening of the RTS makes it easier for the wire to turn into the instrument, whilst the longer posterior lip of the RTS protects the posterior tracheal wall from inadvertent needle lesion (Fig. 9.12).

The large gap between the telescope and the RTS lumen ensures free ventilation. The placement of the rigid tracheoscope, in our experience, raised some difficulties only in a few cases, however, not such as to interrupt the procedure. The retromolar passage of the instrument (Fig. 9.10), greatly facilitated the maneuvre. A useful safety precaution was to achieve a clear vision of the tip of the RTS near the vocal cords before removing the endotracheal tube to ensure a quick substitution. In addition, in the patients with primary difficult intubation or with facial abnormalities, the substitution of the RTS and also of the ventilation catheter was practiced under a tube exchanger protection (Figs 9.27 and 9.28).

With the FFB variation, the trachea is mobile, shifting laterally and down. The whole ETT/FFB system does not ensure enough support to the anterior wall, and so, the tracheal squashing facilitates the perforation of the posterior wall and impairs endoscopic vision, predisposing to ectopic punctures and false passages. Frequently, many punctures are attempted which increase the

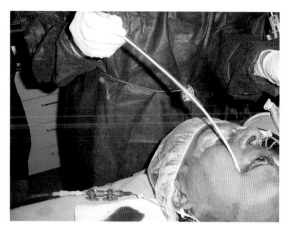

Fig. 9.27: Tube exchanger inside the RTS

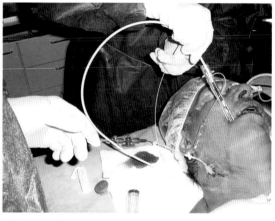

Fig. 9.28: Tube exchanger inside the ventilation-catheter

occurrence of vascular and lung injury remarkably. Another drawback of ETT/FFB is difficult ventilation due to high respiratory resistances. However, the FFB variation could be fitting for particular conditions of difficult airway approach and is recommended in patients with an unstable cervical spine.[4]

Phase 2: It is identical in every kind of TLT. The retrograde, or inside/outside dilation, is the exclusive characteristic of the technique, and therefore, does not have any alternatives. The advantages of the TLT in Phase 2 can be understood by looking at Fig. 9.15. The cone follows a compulsory way

therefore, eliminating the risk of lesion of the posterior tracheal wall, always incumbent in other percutaneous tracheostomies. No other technique can boast a dilatation phase that is so rapid, only a few seconds, and so free from danger that it is feasible to do without endoscopic checking. It is a rare example of a maneuvre with absolute intrinsic safety, non operator-dependent.

In addition, on the contrary with what happens with OITs, where high resistances mean high risk of complications. With TLT it is possible to affirm that there is not a limit for a pulling force and the higher the resistances are the more regular is the stoma. In fact, the opposite pressures of the fingers and cone afford the compacting and blockage of the neck layers so that the cone can pass through them without stretching and jagging the ridge of the stoma. The strong compacting of the tissue, tightly pressed between the fingers and the emerging cone, is the true keynote of the lowest local trauma. Tracheal ring fractures, so frequent especially in single step dilation techniques,[5,6] mucosal flaps and bleedings are almost absent.

TLT is esteemed to be the elective technique for patients with extreme coagulopathies.[7-9] In addition, it is remarkable to notice that over all these years, no mention has been reported of higher rates of stomal or systemic infections, if compared with OITs,[10,11] as one might have expected on the basis of the oral passage of the cannula.

Phase 3: TLT offers the significant advantage of not at all contemplating the introduction of the cannula: it is already inside the airway and only requires to be turned caudally.

In the basic TLT, the telescope placed inside the cannula allows a millimetrical control of the shifting of the internal part of the cannula, making the decannulation quite unlikely. However, during the straightening and the rotation, the cannula may come out of the tracheal lumen if a proper endoscopic control is not practiced. This inconvenience can be easily mended by the insertion of a new cone-cannula, exploiting the safety thread (Fig. 9.29), with the same procedure of the TLT Phase 2.

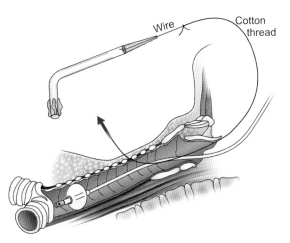

Fig. 9.29: Insertion of a new cone-cannula, using the safety thread

The straightening and rotation of the cannula by means of 0° telescope, are maneuvres which, being unusual, at first seem complex but, after a while, they appear to be simple and easy to learn,[4,12] especially if the clinical practice is preceded by a short training on a dummy, which was built on purpose (Fig. 9.30).

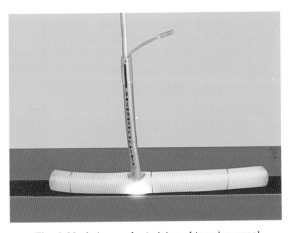

Fig. 9.30: A dummy for training of translaryngeal tracheostomy

Ventilation

In TLT method, both RTS and the ventilation catheter are cuffed and so providing, through a closed respiratory system, high levels of PIP and PEEP as well. In this way it is possible to practice TLT under completely adequate respiratory assistance also in the ALI/ARDS patients.[8,13] An uncuffed small tube is recommended,[14] but obviously, it is not suitable for this kind of patient. The lack of a significant increase of CO_2 enables TLT to be applied also in patients with severe brain damage.[15] Furthermore, the security offered by the presence of the ventilation catheter in Phase 3, when an accidental decannulation might more likely happen, is unquestionable.

Respiratory assistance can be performed with mechanical ventilator or manually, particularly in infants. Manual or mechanical jet ventilation can also be adopted, however is advisable to use this technique exclusively with mechanical ventilator equipped with very sensible alarm's systems. We used manual jet ventilation in few cases [2], but we abandoned this modality of ventilation because when manual control systems are used, there is always the risk of acute pulmonary over-distension and air leak.

Variations that are not Advisable

Three methods, potentially dangerous, are widely diffused because they are quicker and shortcut procedures.

In a few centers the needle is inserted blindly. Even if the users boast that this variation allows a good training in the retrograde intubation technique, otherwise very difficult to reach in normal practice, this method is not advisable because many punctures are frequently required with the resulting increase of tissue trauma, bleeding and risk of pleural lesion.

Some users practice withdrawing the ventilation catheter before the translaryngeal passage of the cone-cannula and accomplish the maneuvres of

Phases 2 and 3 in apnea in the assumption that the presence of the ventilation catheter could interfere with the straightening and rotation of the cannula, but there is a wide gap between the two devices (Fig. 9.31).

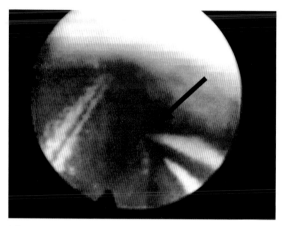

Fig. 9. 31: The arrow shows the wide gap between the cone and the catheter ventilation

Other users skip the endoscopic control in Phase 3. Proceeding in this way, one should not wonder if decannulation, desaturations and hypercapnia then occur.

Programmed Replacement of the Cannula

The cannula supplied with the kit may remain *in situ* for long periods, without problems, thanks to its characteristics and particularly to its flexibility. During the first 24-48 hours, the stoma of the TLT, as that one of OITs, tends to shrink and cannula substitution is not recommended. After 24-48 hours there are not specific problem related to TLT and the cannula can be changed, if necessary, with usual precautions adopted during any cannula replacement and with particular regard to patient anatomy. When the patient is transferred to a general ward or to external rehabilitation wards is essential to change the cannula with one having a counter-cannula.

CASE STUDIES

All the patients admitted in the general ICU of the Community Hospital San Carlo Borromeo, Milan, Italy, from July 1993 to March 1996, with the usual indications for elective tracheostomy were studied. It consists of a first uninterrupted series of 95 adults and 14 children (Table 9.2) who underwent TLT with several modalities[2] and a second uninterrupted series of 302 adults and 12 children, from April 1996 to November 2006 (Table 9.3) in which only the basic TLT technique was adopted at the patient's bedside.

No preliminary exclusion was made of the difficult cases. At least 20% of the patients were either absolutely contra-indicated for percutaneous tracheostomies, such as infants, children and adults without external landmarks, untreatable coagulopathies or severe acute respiratory failure.

In a first series of 109 patients[2] the complications encountered were: one early minor hemorrhage, one pneumothorax without consequences in a patient in manual jet ventilation, three cases of desaturations without consequences due to the prevailing use of apnea method in adults, and three total extractions of the cannula.

In the second series of 314 patients the complications observed were: one early minor hemorrhage, two total extractions of the cannula and two cases desaturations without consequences, caused by a non suitable resetting of the respirator after the insertion of the ventilation catheter, through inadvertence. Arterial samples, obtained after induction of anesthesia, with the patient still intubated, and at the end of Phases 1, 2 and 3 after the placement of the ventilation catheter, generally showed a normal saturation and a CO_2 level stable or even lowered.

In properly ventilated patients there were some fluctuations in arterial blood pressure that resulted to be in strict relationship with the level of anesthesia. The authors didn't encounter any lesions of the posterior tracheal wall in the entire population.

Table 9.2: Characteristics of patients and underlying diseases of the first series (1993-1996)			
Adults			
Total patients	95	COPD	34 (35.8%)
• male	60 (63%)	Cardiac diseases	22 (23.1%)
• female	35 (37%)	Postsurgery	17 (17.9%)
average age (years)	60 ± 11	Neurological diseases	9 (9.5%)
SAPS I	15±3	ALI/ARDS	7 (7.4%)
Timing	11±3	Trauma patients	6 (6.3%)
Infants and Children			
Total patients	14	Neurological patients and central airway obstruction	5 (35.7 %)
• male	9 (64.3%)	Stenosis/malacia	5 (35.7%)
• female	5 (35.7 %)	Cardiac diseases and central airway obstruction	4 (28.6%)
average age (months)	26±18		

Table 9.3: Characteristics of patients and underlying diseases of the second series (1996-2006)			
Adults			
Total patients	302	COPD	120 (40%)
• male	180 (59.6%)	Cardiac diseases	60 (20%)
• female	122 (40.4%)	ALI/ARDS	33 (11%)
average age (years)	68.3 ± 12	Neurological diseases	42 (14%)
SAPS II	50.6 ± 16.2	Trauma patients	24 (8%)
Timing	13.3 ± 8.4	Postsurgery	23 (7%)
Infants and Children			
Total patients	12	Neurological diseases	3 (25 %)
• male	9 (75%)	Stenosis/malacia	3 (25%)
• female	3 (25 %)	ALI/ARDS	3 (25%)
average age (months)	42 ± 38.6	Cardiac diseases	2 (16.66%)
Facial abnormalities	1 (8.34%)		

As regards post procedural complications like late cicatricial narrowing of the trachea, we believe that postoperative nursing may be very determining in addition to the degree of technique-related trauma. However, previous studies[2,16], have not found any stenosis in twenty adult patients submitted to long term follow-up by means of endoscopic control and/or computed tomography. In 9 patients subjected to autopsy at different intervals after tracheostomy, there were some flat, non-infiltrated breaches, without torn tissues or fractured rings. In the second series of 302 adult patients, long term follow-up was made in only 32 cases out of 47 contacts, because of the high percentage of patients transferred, and still cannulated, to external rehabilitation wards. A narrowing was found in two cases, in one patient at the laryngotracheal junction and in the second one in the lower trachea, both far from the stoma and thus, not to be considered closely correlated with the tracheostomy technique.

The technique has been studied by many authors[8,12,17-20] and is deemed an acceptable approach to percutaneous tracheostomy. Westphal et al performed elective TLT in 120 patients and concluded that the technique was safe and cost effective.[19]

Byhahn et al[21] studied Fantoni's TLT technique and Griggs guidewire dilating forceps PDT to evaluate these two techniques in terms of perioperative complications, risks, and benefits in 100 critically ill patients (50 patients in each group). Tracheostomy was performed under general anesthesia at the patient's bedside. The mean (± SD) operating times were short, 9.2 ± 3.9 minutes (TLT) and 4.8 ± 3.7 minutes (GWDF) on average. Perioperative complications were noted in two (4%) of patients during either TLT or GWDF and included massive bleeding, mediastinal emphysema, posterior tracheal wall injury, and pretracheal placement of the tracheostomy tube. In one patient, who developed posterior tracheal wall perforation with TLT technique during intratracheal rotation of tracheostomy tube, conventional surgical tracheostomy was performed by ENT surgeon. No perioperative hypoxia was noted regardless of the technique used. The authors concluded that both TLT and GWDF represent attractive, safe alternatives to conventional tracheostomy or other percutaneous procedures if carefully performed by experienced physicians under bronchoscopic control.

Divisi et al[22] compared the operative technique and complications of the TLT with those of the Ciaglia Blue Rhino tracheostomy (CBR); TLT in 350 and CBR in 120 adult critically ill patients. Ciaglia Blue Rhino tracheostomy was noted to have a cost-benefit advantage over TLT. The CBR tracheostomy took less time to perform and had fewer complications than TLT, because the technique was simpler.

CONCLUSIONS

All the modalities of carrying out TLT have in common an identical Phase 2. The inside-outside direction of the dilation maneuvre offers the great benefit of the complete elimination of the most dangerous complications of the outside-inside percutaneous methods: the tearing of the posterior tracheal wall. A second benefit is represented by the absence of a true insertion of the cannula, as it is atraumatically dragged to the inside of the trachea by the cone, in Phase 2. Also the mechanism of the creation of the two opposite pressures, is determinant in reducing, through a strong compression of the peristomal tissue, the local trauma, the stretching and bleeding. In addition, the pure dilation obtained in this way, ensures an unmatchable adherence of the stoma to the cannula.

For all these exclusive advantages, the TLT method may extend its indications to the contraindications of OITs.

REFERENCES

1. Ciaglia and Fantoni methods. Ann Thorac Surg 1999;68:486-92.
2. Konopke R, Zimmermann T, Volk A, Pirc J, Bergert H, Blomenthal A, Gastmeier J, Kersting S. Prospective evaluation of the retrograde percutaneous Fantoni A. Translaryngeal tracheostomy. In Gullo A. editor APICE Trieste 1993:459-65.
3. Fantoni A, Ripamonti D. A non-derivative, non-surgical tracheostomy: The translaryngeal method. Intensive Care Med 1997;23:386-92.
4. Fantoni A. Nuovi criteri di comparazione: le fasi della tracheostomia e i dati anatomici essenziali. Minerva Anestesiol 2004;70:445-8.
5. Sharpe MD, Parnes LS, Drover JW, Harris C. Translaryngeal tracheostomy: Experience of 340 cases. Laryngoscope 2003;113:530-6.
6. Byhahn C, Wilke HJ, Halbig S, Lischke V, Westphal K. Percutaneous tracheostomy: Ciaglia Blue Rhino versus the basic Ciaglia technique of percutaneous dilational tracheostomy. Anesth Analg 2000;91:882-6.
7. Kinnear JA, Higgins DJ. Tracheal ring fracture and herniation with PercuTwist percutaneous dilator. Intensive Care Med 2004;30:1242-3.
8. MacCallum PL, Parnes LS, Sharpe MD, Harris C. Comparison of open, percutaneous, and translaryngeal tracheostomies. Otolaryngol Head Neck Surg 2000;122:686-90.
9. Byhahn C, Lischke V, Westphal K. Translaryngeal tracheostomy in highly unstable patients. Anaesthesia 2000;55:678-82.
10. Sharpe MD, Parnes LS, Drover JW, Harris C. Translaryngeal tracheostomy: Experience of 340 cases. Laryngoscope 2003;113:530-6.

11. Antonelli M, Michetti V, Di Palma A, Conti G, Pennisi MA, Arcangeli A, Montini L, Bocci MG, Bello G, Almadorui G, Paludetti G, Proietti R. Percutaneous translaryngeal versus surgical tracheostomy: A randomized trial with 1-y double-blind follow-up. Crit Care Med 2005;33:1015-20.

12. Westphal K, Byhahn C, Rinne T, Wilke HJ, Wimmer-Greinecker G, Lischke V. Tracheostomy in cardiosurgical patients. Surgical tracheostomy versus translaryngeal tracheostomy (Fantoni procedure) in a surgical intensive care unit: Technique and results of the Fantoni tracheostomy. Head & Neck 2006;28:355-9.

13. Benini A, Rossi N, Maisano P, Marcolin R, Patroniti N, Pesenti A, Foti G. Translaryngeal tracheostomy in acute respiratory distress syndrome patients. Intensive Care Med 2002;28:726-30.

14. Ferraro F, Capasso A, Troise E, Lanza S, Azan G, Rispoli F, Belluomo Anello C. Assessment of ventilation during the performance of elective endoscopic-guided percutaneous tracheostomy: Clinical evaluation of a new method. Chest 2004;126:159-64.

15. Stocchetti N, Parma A, Songa V, Colombo A, Lamperti M, Tognini L. Early translaryngeal tracheostomy in patient with severe brain damage. Intensive Care Med 2000;26:1101-7.

16. Fantoni A, Ripamonti D, Lesmo A, Zanoni CI. Tracheostomia translaringea. Nuova era? Minerva Anestesiol 1996;62:313-25.

17. Karnik A, Freeman JW. Translaryngeal tracheostomy technique (TLT): Prospective evaluation of 164 cases. Br J Anaesth 1999;82 (suppl 1):169.

18. Vecchiarelli P, et al. Fantoni's translaryngeal tracheostomy: Two years of experience. Br J Anaesth 1999;82 (suppl 1):167.

19. Westphal K, Byhahn C, Rinne T, Wilke HJ, Wimmer-Greinecker G, Lischke V. Tracheostomy in cardiosurgical patients: Surgical tracheostomy versus Ciaglia and fantoni methods. Ann Thor Surg 1999;68:486-92.

20. Westphal K, Byhahn C, Wilke HJ, Lischke V. Percutaneous tracheostomy: A clinical comparison of dilatational (Ciaglia) and translaryngeal (Fantoni) techniques. Anesth Analg 1999;89:938-43.

21. Byhahn C, Wilke HJ, Lischke V, Rinne T, Westphal K. Bedside percutaneous tracheostomy: Clinical comparison of Griggs and Fantoni techniques. World J Surg 2001; 25:296-301.

22. Divisi D, Altamura G, Di Tommaso S, Di Leonardo G, Rosa E, De Sanctis C, Crisci R. Fantoni translaryngeal tracheostomy versus ciaglia blue rhino percutaneous tracheostomy: A retrospective comparison. Surg Today 2009;39:387-92.

Chapter 10

Balloon Facilitated Percutaneous Tracheostomy

Christian Byhahn

INTRODUCTION

All minimally invasive techniques of tracheostomy have two independent steps in common: dilatation of pretracheal tissues and the anterior tracheal wall, and the cannula insertion performed in subsequent order. Only translaryngeal tracheostomy (TLT) is different in that dilatation is achieved with the tracheostomy cannula itself. However, TLT is performed in retrograde, "reverse", fashion, i.e. from inside the trachea to the outside, and is technically quite sophisticated when compared to antegrade techniques. The Griggs technique was reported to have significant major perioperative complications, whereas the Blue Rhino technique showed less severe but still potentially significant perioperative complications.[1-3] Dilatation and cannula placement in separate steps may contribute to some problems and risks. The more manipulation is posed to the airway, the higher is the risk of airway injury, bleeding, creating false passages or entirely loosing the airway. Therefore, it seemed desirable to develop an antegrade tracheostomy technique that combines tracheal dilatation and cannula placement in one single step.

Shortly before his death in 2000 at the age of 88 years, the pioneer of modern percutaneous tracheostomy, Pasquale Ciaglia, came up with an idea of balloon facilitated percutaneous tracheostomy (BFPT), an innovative one-step technique. His preliminary visions were further refined by Michael Zgoda, pulmonologist at the University of Kentucky, Lexington, KY, USA. The basic idea behind BFPT was – like Seldinger's guide wire technique – adopted from radiologists who are using balloon dilation for a variety of interventional procedures for almost ages. This technique utilizes a means of dilatation that does not require entry into the trachea by downward pressure using a hard dilatational device, which theoretically could decrease the risk of posterior tracheal wall injuries.

APPARATUS AND THE PROCEDURE

BFPT combines dilatation and cannula placement in one single step. First, a 15-20 mm longitudinal or horizontal skin incision has to be made. Like with any other minimally-invasive technique, the trachea is then punctured under bronchoscopic vision, and a guidewire is introduced through the needle into the trachea. The needle is withdrawn, and the dilator-cannula device is passed over the guidewire.

The heart of BFPT is a device that can be divided into two portions: the distal portion of the assembly holds a deflated balloon, while the proximal portion is armed with the tracheostomy cannula (Fig. 10.1). In 2003, Michael Zgoda reported on his initial experience with BFPT in four dogs.[4] After skin incision, tracheal puncture and guidewire placement, the puncture channel is pre-dilated with a 14-French punch dilator taken from a Blue Rhino kit. Thereafter, the BFPT device holding a 50 mm long, deflated balloon is passed over the guidewire until the distal portion of the balloon became visible in the trachea. The balloon is now inflated with saline solution to create a pressure of five atmosphere (Fig. 10.2). Such pressure exerted on live tissue results in immediate ischemia. Subsequently, tissue looses its elastic properties. The balloon is left inflated for about 30 seconds, and, lubricated with saline solution, entirely passed down into the trachea thereafter. The puncture canal essentially enlarges with the balloon by outward radial pressure. The proximal portion of the BFPT device that carried the tube is introduced in the trachea, thereby the cannula is placed. The last step is to deflate the balloon by evacuating the saline solution, and to remove apparatus and guidewire through the cannula. The tracheal tube cuff is then inflated and the correct placement of the cannula is verified by

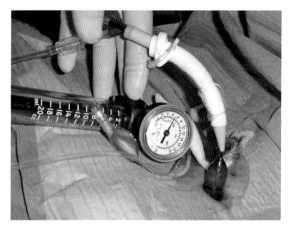

Fig. 10.2: Balloon facilitated percutaneous tracheostomy. An angioplasty balloon is inflated at 5 atm to create a tracheal stoma. After balloon deflation the device is advanced further into the trachea and the tracheostomy cannula placed thereby

bronchoscopy. The ventilator is then connected to the tracheostomy tube and the orotracheal tube is removed.

Like almost any other invention, the BFPT device underwent various modifications, both in design and technique itself, on its way from the animal laboratory to the bedside.[5-7] One reason was that advancing the inflated balloon completely into the trachea appeared to be difficult in some cases, despite proper lubrication. Another concern was the potential risk of bronchial injury if the device was introduced relatively too deep in smaller persons. Therefore, Zgoda successfully tested a technique of deflating the balloon before pushing it down the trachea. Ischemic preconditioning of the cervical tissues makes the dilated stoma stay open long enough to introduce the cannula, even if the blood flow has returned in the meantime. It takes about seconds before previously ischemic tissue retrieves its elastic properties and such the ability to contract – enough time to advance the cannula.

In the meantime, a couple of cases have been published on the feasibility of BFPT in humans.[8] In most cases, cannula placement was successful in the first attempt, but sometimes re-inflation of

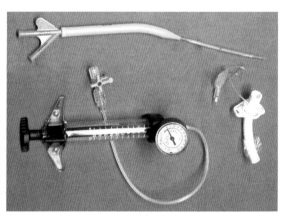

Fig. 10.1: Balloon dilatation percutaneous tracheostomy kit

the balloon was required to enhance the quality of dilatation. A reason for this could have been different elastic properties of the cervical tissues, i.e. fat or muscle have little resistance to five atmosphere of balloon pressure and is dilated instantly, while the cervical fascia is tougher and thus more difficult to dilate. Uneven resistance alongside of the inflated balloon can create an hour-glass effect that results in uneven pressure distribution within the balloon. The operator, in turn, measures an overall balloon pressure which does not necessarily reflect the actual pressure in a particular area of the balloon. Despite sufficient overall balloon pressure, insufficient pressure at a particular point (i.e. fascia) results in insufficient dilation and thus inability to introduce the cannula. Using a balloon with higher rated burst pressure (e.g. 10-15 atmosphere) could be an option to solve this problem.

Another technical problem of BFPT is balloon rupture before full dilation is achieved. Zgoda, in laboratory investigations, could show that the balloon typically bursts at the narrowest portion of the hour-glass, which, in turn, is typically the site of the least degree of dilatation. When this happened in one patient, attempted removal of the ruptured balloon catheter through the stoma caused crimping of the distal half of the balloon forming a button within the airway and preventing removal.[9] A recovery procedure has therefore been developed. Zgoda demonstrated during induced balloon ruptures in cadavers, that advancement of the device into the airway to exploit the loading dilator to further dilate the stoma and allow balloon catheter removal was successful. The wire remained in place and allowed placement of another device and successful tracheostomy.

One of the important clinical considerations related to this procedure is temporary occlusion of trachea with the balloon for about at least for 15 seconds. Thus in the susceptible patients apnea for such period may evoke life-threatening hypoxemia.

Therefore, balloon dilatation technique may not be a good choice for that individual.[7]

Recently, Gromann et al[10] reported their experience of balloon dilatational tracheostomy using the Ciaglia Blue Dolphin Set (Ciaglia Blue Dolphin Balloon Percutaneous Tracheostomy Introducer, Cook Critical Care, Bloomington, IN, USA) in 20 patients from a cardiosurgical intensive care unit. The surgical time was 3.3 ± 1.9 min. No significant bleeding or tracheal wall injury was observed; however, there were two complications. One patient developed single tracheal ring cartilage fracture and other subcutaneous emphysema during the balloon dilatation. The study concluded that balloon dilatational tracheostomy is feasible, easy, and safe in the hands of experienced users.

CONCLUSION

The BFPT represents the first antegrade one-step tracheostomy device. In animal and cadaver studies the technique proved feasible and technically simple. A few published cases in patients mainly confirmed these findings. Nevertheless, large and comparative clinical trials need to be conducted before a final statement regarding clinical impact of this novel technique can be made.

REFERENCES

1. Ambesh SP, Pandey CK, Srivastava S, Agarwal A, Singh DK. Percutaneous tracheostomy with single dilatation technique: A prospective, randomized comparison of Ciaglia blue rhino versus Griggs guidewire dilating forceps. Anesth Analg 2002;95:1739-45.
2. Fikkers BG, Briede IS, Verwiel JM, et al. Percutaneous tracheostomy with the Blue Rhino trade mark technique: Presentation of 100 consecutive patients. Anaesthesia 2002;57:1094-7.
3. Anon JM, Escuela MP, Gomez V, et al. Percutaenous tracheostomy: Ciaglia Blue Rhino versus Griggs' guide wire dilating forceps: A prospective randomized trial. Acta Anaesthesiol Scand 2004;48:451-6.
4. Zgoda M, Berger R. Balloon facilitated percutaneous tracheostomy tube placement: A novel technique. Chest 2003;124:130S-1S.

5. Zgoda M, deBoisblanc B, Berger R. Balloon facilitated percutaneous dilational tracheostomy: A human cadaver feasibility study. Chest 2004;126:735S.

6. Zgoda M, deBoisblanc B, Byhahn C. Balloon facilitated percutaneous dilational tracheostomy: Entire experience of this novel technique. Proc Am Thorac Soc 2005;2:A439.

7. Zgoda M, Berger R. Balloon facilitated percutaneous dilational tracheostomy tube placement: Preliminary report of a novel technique. Chest 2005;128:3688-90.

8. Zgoda M, Byhahn C. Balloon facilitated percutaneous tracheostomy: Does it really work? Intensive Care Med 2005;31:A146.

9. Zgoda MA, deBoisblanc BP. Technique for removal of ruptured balloon catheter occurring during balloon facilitated percutaneous tracheostomy tube placement. Eur Respir J 2005;26 (Suppl 49):533s.

10. Gromann TW, Birkelbach O, Hetzer R. Balloon dilatational tracheostomy: Technique and first clinical experience with the Ciaglia Blue Dolphin method. Chirung 2008; Dec.4.

Chapter 11

Percutaneous Dilatational Tracheostomy with Ambesh T-Trach Kit

Chandra Kant Pandey

INTRODUCTION

Introduction of Ciaglia's multiple sequential dilators percutaneous tracheostomy kit,[1] in 1985, has led to the rejuvenation of interest in the percutaneous dilational tracheostomy (PDT). In 1999, Ciaglia developed single flexible Rhino's horn like dilator 'Ciaglia Blue Rhino' and announced that the rigid dilators were too dangerous and thus, they must be banned. He wrote: "The day of the rigid dilators in PDT, curved or straight, is over. No matter what rigid dilator they are using, that the rigid, straight, or curved dilator, inserted at right angles, can still cause trauma to the posterior tracheal wall if too much force is exerted."[2]

Now a days, PDT has become one of the most commonly performed minimally invasive surgical procedures in intensive care unit patients. Various PDT kits are available for clinical use[1,3-7] and each has been claimed to have some advantages over the others. Recently, a percutaneous dilatational tracheostomy introducer kit "T-Trach" (manufactured by Eastern Medikit Limited, 196 Phase-I, Udyog Vihar Gurgaon-122016, India), has been introduced to facilitate the formation of bedside PDT. In fact, the T-Trach is a rechristened name of the Ambesh

T-Dagger (Criticure Invasives, India) that was initially introduced in the year 2005 [8-10] but was withdrawn due to manufacture dispute.

The T-Trach is a T-shaped, semi-rigid device made up of polyvinyl chloride (Fig. 11.1). The shaft of the T-Trach is smoothly curved at an angle of about 30°, elliptical in cross section and has a number of oval holes. These holes are intended to provide to-and-fro airflow during ventilation when the shaft lay inside the tracheal lumen during stoma formation. The shaft of the T-Trach, due to its elliptical shape, should leave enough space in tracheal lumen and thereby decreases the risk of air trapping into the lungs. The proximal end of the device is incorporated with a 5 cm long guide catheter while the distal end has two shoulders to provide a better grip. The device has a central tunnel to accommodate a guide wire. A well lubricated T-Trach dilator can be inserted over a tracheal guide wire to facilitate tracheal stoma formation. The inherent design of the device should form adequate size of tracheal stoma by splitting the space between two tracheal rings, when inserted until its base touches the skin and distal black mark lay inside the trachea, while avoiding an over-dilatation of tracheal stoma.

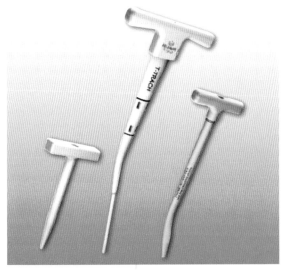

Percutaneous Tracheostomy Kit (Sterile) Contains:

- Surgical blade
- Tracheal puncture cannula on needle
- Syringes (5 ml and 10 ml)
- Guidewire
- 14 FG initial dilator
- T-trach dilator
- Lubricating jelly
- Tracheostomy tube introducer
- Hemostat
- Gauze pieces

Fig. 11.1: (left to right): Initial dilator, T-Trach dilator and tracheostomy tube introducer
(*Courtesy:* Eastern Medikit Limited, India)

PROCEDURAL STEPS

The steps of formation of percutaneous tracheostomy with the T-Trach are essentially the same as with Ciaglia's Blue Rhino (CBR) percutaneous dilatational tracheostomy technique that uses Seldinger guide wire. The only difference is that the introduction of separate guide catheter is not required. The contraindications include emergency tracheostomy, local sepsis, enlarged thyroid, pediatric patients (less than 12 years), difficult unprotected airway, stenosis of upper airway, severe coagulopathies, unstable cervical spine fracture, high PEEP (>20 cm.H_2O) and extreme circulatory insufficiency. Routine patient monitoring includes: continuous electrocardiography, arterial blood pressure, peripheral hemoglobin oxygen saturation (SpO_2), end-tidal carbon dioxide ($EtCO_2$) and peak airway pressure (PAP). All patients should receive general anesthesia along with relaxant to facilitate controlled ventilation on 100% oxygen. Position the patient supine with moderate extension of neck, as for conventional surgical tracheostomy, by placing a small wedge beneath the shoulders. Perform the fiberoptic bronchoscopy, visualize the trachea and carina and withdraw the endotracheal

tube until the tip of the tube lay immediately above the vocal cords. Aseptic preparation of the neck is done and thyroid cartilage, cricoid cartilage, suprasternal notch and intended tracheostomy site (preferably between tracheal rings 2-3) are marked. If the tracheal rings are not palpable then a midpoint between the cricoid cartilage and suprasternal notch may be selected. About 10 ml of lignocaine (1%) with adrenaline (1: 200,000) is injected at this site to prevent oozing from the subcutaneous tissue.

The trachea is stabilized with thumb and index finger of one hand and a 1 cm long transverse skin incision is made at the intended tracheostomy site. Following the skin incision, though not mandatory, it is advised to dissect the pretracheal tissues with a pair of curved mosquito forceps. Under fiberoptic bronchoscopic guidance, anterior tracheal wall is punctured with a 14-gauge cannula-on-needle and tracheal entry of the cannula is confirmed on aspiration of air into the saline-filled syringe and by direct bronchoscopic visualization of cannula into the tracheal lumen. A "J" tip guide wire is inserted through the cannula towards the carina until about 20 cm. The cannula is removed and a 14-French well lubricated initial dilator is advanced over the guide wire in order to start a tracheal stoma formation. Now the T-Trach dilator, with its shaft well lubricated, is loaded over the guide wire and advanced slowly into the trachea at an angle of about 90° until the proximal mark lay inside. Free movement of the guide wire through the T-Trach must be ensured. The direction of the T-Trach dilator is then changed to about 60° angle and advanced further until its base touches the skin and the distal black mark lay inside the tracheal lumen. After formation of tracheal stoma the T-Trach dilator is removed leaving the guide wire *in situ*. A well lubricated cuffed tracheostomy tube loaded on its introducer/obturator over the guide wire and inserted through the tracheal stoma. Following placement of the tracheostomy tube tracheal suction is performed, the tracheal cuff is inflated, and ventilation of lungs is resumed through the tracheostomy tube (Figs 11.2A to F). The

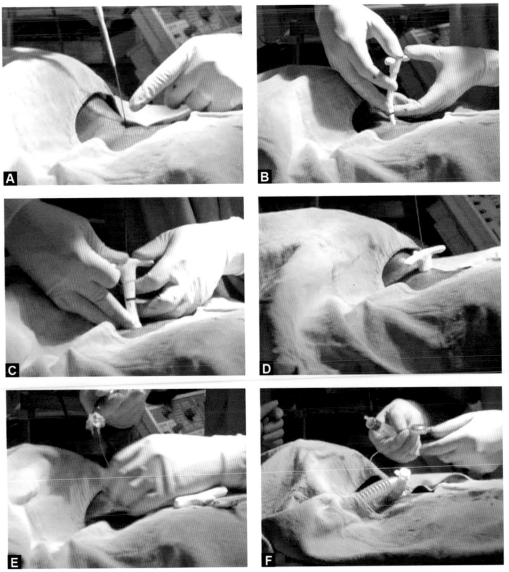

Figs 11.2A to F: Following placement of the guide wire tracheal dilatation and insertion of tracheostomy tube with T-Trach

endotracheal tube is removed once the ventilation of lungs through the tracheostomy tube is ensured.

Air entry into the lungs must be confirmed by respiratory plethysmography and $EtCO_2$ and correct placement of tracheostomy tube by bronchoscopy. The neck and chest should be palpated to exclude development of surgical emphysema. At the end of the procedure chest X-ray should be requested to locate distal end of the tracheostomy tube and to exclude development of pneumothorax and surgical emphysema.

In initial evaluations, the T-Trach has been found successful in formation of bedside PDT. Average procedural time (skin incision to placement of tracheostomy tube) has varied from 3-5 minutes in most of the patients.[8-12] The T-Trach has provided appropriate size of tracheal stoma for the corresponding size of tracheostomy tube with no under or over dilatation. It has not been associated with difficulty in its insertion, restricted bronchoscopic view during stoma dilatation, hemorrhage, tracheal injury, pneumothorax or increased airway resistance to compromise ventilation. The elliptical shape of the shaft forms the tracheal stoma by splitting intertracheal ring membrane and has not been associated with tracheal rings fracture and invagination of stoma margins into the tracheal lumen. Short procedural time and insignificant increase in peak airway pressure may be advantageous when the procedure is performed in patients who require a high inspired oxygen concentration and have stiff lungs.

A prospective and comparative study has shown superior results in comparison to Ciaglia Blue Rhino.[8] The authors have demonstrated that while forming tracheal stoma with the CBR about three-fourth of the tracheal lumen is occluded resulting into significant increase in peak airway pressure while it was not so with the T-Trach dilator. Further, the cephalad tracheal ring is vulnerable for fracture due to transmitted pressure exerted during introduction of the CBR.[12] These findings are

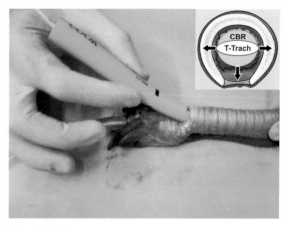

Fig. 11.3: Showing near total occlusion of the lumen of sheep trachea with Ciaglia Blue Rhino (CBR). Inset showing comparison of CBR (blue) with T-Trach dilator (white)

corroborated while forming the PDT in a sheep trachea model (Fig. 11.3).

CONCLUSION

The T-Trach PDT kit facilitates formation of PDT and shows an initial promise as an alternative device to Ciaglia's Blue Rhino. The device has been claimed to be superior to CBR; however, the experience is limited. Prospective, controlled clinical trials with large patient population are awaited to prove its merits over much commonly used CBR kit.

REFERENCES

1. Ciaglia P, Firsching R, Syniec C. Elective percutaneous dilatational tracheostomy. A new simple bedside procedure: Preliminary report. Chest 1985;87:715-9.
2. Ciaglia P. Technique, complications, and improvements in percutaneous dilatational tracheostomy. Chest 1999.
3. Griggs WM, Worthley LIG, Gillgan JE, et al. A simple percutaneous tracheostomy technique. Surg Gynecol Obstetrics 1990;170:543-5.
4. Fantoni A, Ripamonti D. A non-derivative, non-surgical tracheostomy: The translaryngeal method. Intens Care Med 1997;23:386-92.
5. Zgoda M, Berger R. Balloon facilitated percutaneous tracheostomy tube placement: A novel technique. Chest 2003;124:130S-1S.

6. Bewsher M, Adams A, Clarke C, McConachie I, Kelly D. Evaluation of a new percutaneous dilatational tracheostomy set. Anaesthesia 2001;56:859-64.

7. Frova G, Quintel M. A new simple method for percutaneous tracheostomy: Controlled rotating dilation. Intensive Care Med 2002;28:299-303.

8. Ambesh SP, Pandey CK, Tripathi M, Pant KC, Singh PK. Formation of bedside percutaneous tracheostomy with the T-Dagger: A prospective randomized and comparative evaluation with the Ciaglia Blue Rhino. Anesthesiology 2005;103: A316.

9. Ambesh SP, Tripathi M, Pandey CK, Pant KC, Singh PK. Clinical evaluation of the "T-Dagger": A new bedside percutaneous dilational tracheostomy device. Anaesthesia 2005;60:708-11.

10. Ambesh SP, Pandey CK. Ambesh's T-Dagger- A New Device for Quick Bedside Percutaneous Dilational Tracheostomy. Anesth Analg 2005;101:302-3.

11. Gautam SKS, Singh DK. Percutaneous tracheostomy: Ambesh T-Dagger vs Ciaglia Blue Rhino. Annual Conference of Indian Society of Critical Care Medicine 2006.

12. Hooda P, Kaushal AK. T-Trach dilator is superior to Ciaglia Blue Rhino in formation of Percutaneous dilatational tracheostomy: A sheep trachea model study. Animal Model Exp 2007;3:9-11.

Chapter 12

Anesthetic and Technical Considerations for Percutaneous Tracheostomy

Sushil P Ambesh

Percutaneous dilatational tracheostomy (PDT) is gaining in popularity among critical care physicians as an effective means of airway management in patients requiring long-term ventilatory support in the ICU and respiratory rehabilitation facilities.[1] Many studies have advocated PT as a safe, efficient, and cost effective alternative to surgical tracheostomy. Several methods of PT are available as described in earlier chapters; however, all are based on Seldinger guide wire technique.

Before planning for PDT, it is very much prudent to find out whether there is definite indication of tracheostomy and there is no absolute contraindication of the procedure. The contraindications of PT are described elsewhere in this book. It is also important to weigh the reported mortality (0.5-1%) and serious morbidity (5-10%) associated with the PDT against the prospective advantages. Such risks must be taken in consideration and balanced against the risks of translaryngeal intubation and continued use of sedatives and other analgesics. When learning PDT it is important to choose patients who have apparently normal anatomy, coagulation profile and cardiorespiratory stability. With the increased experience it can be performed successfully in more difficult patients.

Though there are many relative contraindications of the PDT; however, some of these may be curtailed depending on the settings of ICU, type of PDT kit to be used and the experience of the operator. As PDT is an elective procedure, it should be performed preferably during normal working hours of the day to ensure timely help from senior anesthetic, surgical or any other speciality staff, in the event of complication.

The procedure must be explained to the patient (if conscious and fully awake) and/or his close relatives; and written consent/assent must be obtained for record. Often, the patient requiring tracheostomy may not be able to sign the consent but may be able to understand verbal or written explanation (sometimes diagrammatic illustration) about what is going to happen. Many a times patient or his/her relatives think that tracheostomy is the treatment of the disease and after getting tracheostomy done the patient will be fine. Therefore, it is important to explain that tracheostomy is not the treatment of the disease per se; however, formation of tracheostomy may help in facilitating the artificial ventilation, care of respiratory tract or weaning off the ventilator. Further, option of both type of tracheostomy (standard surgical vs percutaneous technique) should be discussed with advantages and disadvantages of each technique before opting for the PDT; and the same should be documented in notes. Such a discussion with patient or relatives provides an ideal opportunity to assess and discuss overall chances of survival, plans of weaning and further care.

The PDT technique should be individualized on the basis of patient parameters. An important consideration related to balloon facilitated percutaneous dilational tracheostomy is that the trachea will become temporarily occluded for 10 to 15 seconds. Three to 5 seconds are required to inflate the balloon, and then another 5-10 seconds of tracheal occlusion are needed to slide the tracheostomy tube into place. Thus, in the unlikely event that 15 seconds of apnea can evoke life-threatening hypoxemia in a given patient, balloon facilitated dilational tracheostomy would not be the procedure of choice for that individual.[2] In the event of laceration of a relatively large blood vessel during the placement of tracheostomy tube with this technique, intraoperative control of the bleeding is not immediately feasible since access to the damaged vessel is limited by the lack of soft tissue.[3]

Presence of anterior jugular vein at the site of intended percutaneous tracheostomy is one of the contraindication. If this vessel is punctured or lacerated during the procedure, it bleeds heavily. The presence of anterior jugular vein or any other vasculature at the site of intended tracheostomy can be diagnosed with the use of ultrasonography or bronchoscopic trans-illumination or trach-light. In author's personal experience, a head down tilt with moderate sustained pressure for about 10 seconds in right hypochondrium makes anterior jugular vein distended and visible, if present. This is a very simple and inexpensive test.

General Preparation

1. Perform full blood coagulation profile (Prothrombin time, activated clotting time, INR and platelets count). A platelet count of >75000 and INR of <1.5 is desirable. If there are correctable coagulation abnormalities then correct them before performing this elective procedure.
2. Obtain written informed consent/assent from the patient or next of kin
3. Withhold heparin prophylaxis at least 12 hours before the procedure
4. Stop continuous hemofiltration about 4-6 hours before the procedure. Wait for about 12 hours after the hemodialysis, if carried out.
5. Stop nasogastric feed at least 4 hours before and aspirate gastric contents just before the procedure
6. Look whether an experienced help from your colleagues (physician or surgeon) is available, if required.
7. Assess and anticipate the potential difficulties or complications and be ready for plan-B

AIRWAY MANAGEMENT DEVICES

Translaryngeal Endotracheal Tube

The most commonly practiced airway maintenance device during formation of percutaneous tracheostomy is cuffed endotracheal tube. The reasons for its wide acceptance are: (1) Most of the patients are already intubated before going for tracheostomy (2) Cuffed endotracheal tube provides proper seal against aspiration (3) The patient can continue to receive PEEP and desired alveolar ventilation without leak. Before formation of PT one of the major requirements is to deflate the cuff and pull back the ET tube into the laryngeal inlet under direct vision to avoid impalement of either the ET tube or its cuff with the tracheal puncture needle or dilators and to leave the intended tracheostomy site free for instrumentation.[4] Even with such a practice, however, cuff perforations and lacerations have been reported.[5] This is not surprising as anatomic length of the adult larynx varies from approximately 3.4-4.4 cm and is also affected by extension and relaxation of neck.[6] Since the average size-8 ET tube cuff length is 3 cm and length of the tube distal to the cuff also measures approximately 3 cm, it is conceivable that with a subcricoid needle puncture, damage of cuff or impalement of tube may occur.[4] A second option is to inflate the cuff above the vocal cords where a gentle pressure is required to achieve a satisfactory seal against the epiglottis, aryepiglottic folds, and the inter-arytenoid fissure to ventilate the lungs.[7]

Care should be taken to prevent aspiration of oral or gastric contents during deflation of ET cuff and adjustment of ET tube. Perform a thorough check-up of the upper airway to predict potential difficulty in translaryngeal re-intubation. Sometimes, patients suffer with severe glottic edema due to prolonged intubation or hypoproteinemia that may make the re-intubation difficult. The tube must be pulled back and repositioned under direct vision using either the laryngoscope or bronchoscope. Though the ideal instrument remains the fiberoptic bronchoscope; the air passage may be protected by using Frova's bougie or airway exchange catheter that may be passed through ET tube until the distal end passes at least 5-10 cm beyond the distal end of the ET tube. Alternatively, a size 14-French suction catheter may be inserted through the top flap hole of catheter mount.[8] This may serve as a tool to prevent inadvertent dislodgement of ET tube as well as for suctioning during the procedure. In the event of accidental loss of airway the ET tube may be rail-roaded over it into the trachea or may be used for insufflation of oxygen.

Supraglottic Airway Devices

Some workers have recommended the removal of ET tube altogether and replacement with laryngeal mask airway (LMA)[9,10] Pro-Seal LMA[11] or intubating LMA[12] provided that the patient is not requiring high inflation pressure or higher fractional inspired oxygen concentration (FiO$_2$ > 60%) or high PEEP (>10 cm H$_2$O) for ventilation. The LMA or its variants make intended tracheostomy site free

of airway device and allows unhindered instrumentation for percutaneous tracheostomy. The large bore of LMA also allows easy ventilation even when fiberoptic bronchoscope is *in situ.* Further, the use of LMA may minimize the risk of damage to the bronchoscope during tracheal puncture.[13] However, one prospective and comparative study[14] has questioned the usefulness of LMA during PT as it was associated with loss of airway and gastric air-distension /regurgitation/ aspiration of gastric contents in number of patients. The device should not be used in patients who are at even little risk of aspiration or airway pressures are more than 20 cm H$_2$O. The study enforces to continue the use of ET tube for this purpose until some better or suitable alternative airway device is available. Other studies have found similar ventilation in both groups[15] or more effective ventilation with the LMA, as evaluated by blood gas analysis.[10]

Cuffed oropharyngeal airway (COPA) (Fig. 12.1) has also been used successfully to maintain the airway during formation of percutaneous tracheostomy.[16,17] However, in a study by Kaya et al, LMA faired better than COPA,[17] where the airway intervention required to maintain patent airway was found to be higher in the COPA group

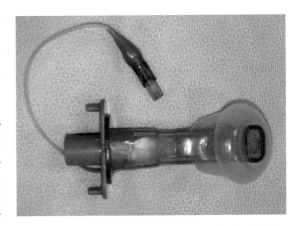

Fig. 12.1: Cuffed oroopharyngeal airway (Mallinckrodt Medical Inc, USA)

(45.2%) than in the LMA group (11.4%). We believe that the applicability and safety of the LMA or COPA in ICU patients, some of whom require high degrees of ventilatory support, are questionable. With the evidence currently available, one can not draw a firm conclusion.

Esophageal Obturator Device: Combitube

A number of case reports have been published with the use of combitube (Fig. 12.2) during percutaneous tracheostomy;[18-20] however, the device has been associated with complications such as esophageal perforation and dilatation.[19] Mallick et al, have noticed significant distortion of airway that posed difficulty in percutaneous tracheostomy and have not recommended its routine use for this procedure.[20]

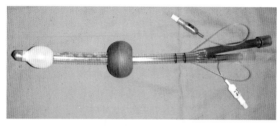

Fig. 12.2: Combitube: Esophageal tracheal double lumen airway (Kendall Sheridan Health Care Products Company, Argyle, NY, USA)

Anesthetic Preparation and Technique

At least, two trained persons are needed; one to manage the airway and other to perform the procedure. If PT is planned under bronchoscopic guidance (preferred if not recommended in all cases) then third person may also be needed. Adequate preoxygenation and optimal positioning of the patient, with moderate extension of head and neck, are followed by surgical disinfection and sterile covering of the operative area. The patient is usually administered 100% FiO_2 on pressure support ventilation under general anesthesia. It is very important that the person looking after the

airway must focus on his job of airway management and monitoring of vitals. Dislodgement of translaryngeal tube or other airway devices during formation of tracheostomy is not uncommon. A loss of airway during middle of the procedure may be life-threatening. Therefore, the task of airway management should not be left to a little experienced anesthesia or intensive care trainee. We suggest following sequence of steps:

- Study the anatomy of neck and potential airway difficulty of the proposed patient. Morbidly obese patients with thick short neck are relative contraindication for PT; however if PT is done in such patients then Ciaglia's method may be preferred over other methods (the author has experienced difficulty in such patients with Griggs or PercuTwist method).

- Select the preferred techniques of percutaneous tracheostomy and kit depending on the experience of operator and general built of the patient.

- Check and keep ready a list of necessary resuscitation equipments and drugs for use in emergency situation.

- Connect a bag of intravenous fluid (preferably a colloid volume expander) for rapid intravenous infusion as most ICU patients after induction of anesthesia tend to develop some degree of hypotension.

- Induce anesthesia with a suitable intravenous anesthetic agent and short acting narcotic. Generally, a combination of propofol, fentanyl and midazolam is quite suitable in a patient who is hemodynamically stable. After induction of anesthesia maintain propofol infusion at a rate of 15-20 ml/hour until completion of the procedure. Etomidate instead of propofol is a better choice for patients who are receiving inotropic or vasopressor support.

- A non-depolarising neuromuscular blocking agent (Atracurium or vecuronium) is administered to facilitate laryngoscopy/ bronchoscopy and ET tube adjustment.

- FiO_2 is increased to 1. Ventilator setting is changed to deliver a tidal volume of about 7-10 ml/kg and minute volume to attain desired $EtCO_2$. The author prefers pressure support ventilation with a PEEP of 5 cm H_2O.
- Once the patient is paralyzed and hemodynamically stable in supine position, place a rolled pillow or sand bag beneath the shoulders to make the neck moderately extended and anatomically landmarks easily identifiable.
- Perform direct laryngoscopy and oropharyngeal suctioning. Assess any potential difficulty of re-intubation. The author is in the habit of keeping a same size and one size smaller ET tubes ready for replacement, if necessary.
- Under direct laryngoscopy, pullback the ET tube until proximal end of the cuff is visible. Hold the tube there with mild inward pressure to prevent it being completely slipping out. Alternatively, a supraglottic airway device may be used to replace the ET tube, wherever appropriate.
- Insert the fiberoptic bronchoscope through flap hole of the catheter mount and ensure its tip lay just at the tip of ET tube (protected within the tube). There is a danger of getting bronchoscope fiber damaged with the tracheal puncture needle or dilator, if tip protrudes beyond the ET Tube. Alternatively, trachlight, bougie or a suction catheter may be used to stabilize the ET tube (Fig. 12.3).

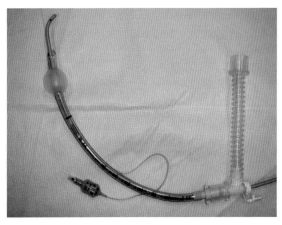

Fig. 12.3: Frova's bougie is placed through flap hole of catheter mount and 15 mm connector

Surgical Preparation and Techniques of PT

Once the patient is anesthetised, paralyzed and hemodynamically stable; tracheostomy position is made. Neck is inspected and palpated for venous and arterial pulsation. A moderate sustained pressure for 10 seconds in right hypochondrium, some times, makes the anterior neck veins visible. Make sure no visible or palpable vessel is coming in the field of intended tracheostomy site. Examine the thickness and length of the neck to choose a proper size of tracheostomy tube. Some manufactures of PT kits provide tracheostomy tube inside the pack, assess whether the provided tracheostomy tube will suit your patient or not. If needed, keep appropriate tracheostomy tube of desired size and length ready.

- Examine the plain chest X-ray for narrowing or deviation of trachea, presence of intrathoracic goitre or any other abnormalities. Many a times, ultrasonography of neck is quite helpful in identifying structures at risk for hemorrhage, such as aberrant blood vessels.[21] Some workers routinely use ultrasonography during tracheal puncture. The relationship between the larynx and the great vessels is inconstant, and damage to the latter during percutaneous tracheostomy with a fatal outcome has been reported.[22] Variant arterial anatomy is well recognized in the neck. Usually, the right subclavian artery is one of the two branches of the right brachiocephalic trunk (innominate artery), the other being the right common carotid artery. In its first part, the subclavian artery ascends about 20 mm above the sternoclavicular joint. But in cadavers, it has been found as high as 40 mm above the joint before arching behind scalenus anterior.[23] It can also arise from below the sternoclavicular joint. A detailed description on ultrasound guided percutaneous tracheostomy can be found elsewhere in this book.

- The operator should scrub, wear sterile gown and gloves. Prepare the neck and upper half of the chest with antiseptic cleansing solutions (povidine iodine and alcohol) and drape the part with sterile surgical drapes.
- Identify/mark the suprasternal notch, thyroid cartilage, cricoid cartilage, and 2nd and 3rd tracheal rings. The most preferred side of tracheostomy is between 2nd and 3rd tracheal rings; however, some workers choose the space between 1st and 2nd or 3rd and 4th tracheal rings. Tracheostomy between cricoid cartilage and 1st tracheal ring should be avoided as it is associated with higher incidence of tracheal stenosis. Further, tracheostomy below the 3rd ring has potential risk of puncturing the great vessels or the highly vascular thyroid isthmus leading to profuse bleeding. If tracheal rings are not palpable then a point between cricoid cartilage and suprasternal notch may be chosen. Occasionally, in obese patients with short neck, the cricoid cartilage may not be palpable; in such patients the author has performed percutaneous tracheostomy just above the suprasternal notch in a number of patients without any untoward incident.
- Infiltrate local anesthetic solution (8-15 ml of lignocaine 1%) with adrenaline (1:200,000) at and around the puncture site to minimize bleeding. Due care must be taken to avoid intravascular injection. A head-up tilt of about 30° helps in reducing the distension of neck veins and bleeding.
- Make a skin incision (1-1.5 cm) at the selected site. Though most authors prefer horizontal incision but the author has not found significant difference between the horizontal or vertical incision. If you have chosen to use vertical incision then it is prudent to stabilize the trachea between thumb and forefingers to ensure midline incision. In author's experience the vertical incision is better in obese patients with obscure anatomical landmarks.
- Though it is debatable to perform blunt dissection of pre-tracheal tissues in a transverse plane with the help of a pair of curved mosquito forceps; however, the author has found it very helpful in identifying arterial pulsation and avoiding puncture of blood vessels. Further, it helps in palpating the position of trachea in midline and tracheal rings with a little finger before making the tracheal puncture. Blunt dissection also helps in reducing the forces required to insert subsequent dilators and tracheostomy tube. Other workers only incise the skin; without dissection of superficial muscle layers, and go on creating the tracheal stoma.
- Tracheal puncture with a cannula on needle, in midline, is guided by digital palpation of trachea or transillumination of tissues with the bronchoscope (Fig. 12.4). As soon as needle enters the tracheal lumen a sudden give way of resistance is felt. The needle entry into the tracheal lumen is confirmed by aspiration of air in saline filled syringe and $EtCO_2$ wave form.

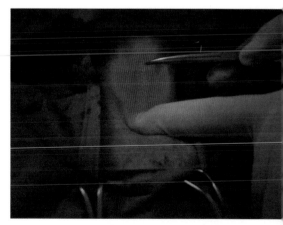

Fig. 12.4: Transillumination of trachea

Aspiration of tracheal mucous is another sign of correct placement of needle in tracheal lumen. Occasionally, needle may be placed in the lung or cuff of the ET tube; and aspiration of air may give a pseudo-impression of needle in the trachea. However, puncture of the ET cuff is easily noticed by sudden fall in airway pressure and activation of low pressure alarm due to air-leak. There are chances of hitting or impaling the ET tube with the needle and that can be detected by asking the person who is managing the airway to gently move the ET tube. In the event of tube impalement a gentle movement of ET tube will move the puncture needle as well. It is possible that the needle may have gone through the Murphy's eye of ET tube (Fig. 12.5) where even gentle movements of ET tube may not detect needle misplacement. Therefore, a direct visualization of needle in tracheal lumen with the help of bronchoscope is highly recommended.

While inserting the tracheal needle/cannula it is important to keep its direction about 60° and caudad so that subsequent passage of guide-wire should not be misplaced upwards. The guide wire must go towards carina to enter in one of the bronchi. This is a very important step of this procedure and therefore it is strongly recommended to confirm the correct placement of guide wire in caudal direction.

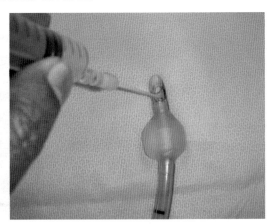

Fig. 12.5: Misplacement of tracheal puncture needle through Murphy's eye

Almost all the procedures of percutaneous tracheostomy have common steps of tracheal puncture and inserting the guide wire. Following placement of guidewire the dilatation of stoma may be initiated and the process may differ a little depending on the type of technique/kit used (Ciaglia's dilators, Griggs Forceps, Frova's PercuTwist, Ambesh T-Trach or Ciaglia's Dolphin balloon). While passing the dilators over the guide wire, the operator must be careful to not to damage posterior tracheal wall which is a soft, muscular structure and quite vulnerable for perforation. During the course of dilatation if operator encounters severe bleeding or desaturation of hemoglobin it is advised to insert the ET tube and place the ET tube cuff at the site of tracheal puncture to create balloon tamponade. Control the bleeding with external pressure or hemostat and decide whether to proceed further or seek experienced help. Never make prestige issue in seeking an experienced help whenever you are in trouble, as little hesitancy on your part may jeopardise the life of an innocent patient. A details description of each technique is given in respective chapters of this book.

Insertion of Tracheostomy Tube and Verification

Some kits include the tracheostomy tube while others not. Therefore, a tracheostomy tube of chosen size and length is lubricated with aqueous jelly after testing its cuff and loaded on a provided introducer/obturator. While choosing the size of the tracheostomy tube one must remember that it should not be too big or too small. Practically, there is no significant advantage of selecting a tracheostomy tube bigger than 9 mm (inner diameter); however, tube size less than 7 mm will have more resistance in air flow and is prone for frequent blockage with thick tracheal secretions.

While introducing the tracheostomy tube the operator must not exert excessive pressure. If tube insertion is too tight then better to dilate tracheal stoma a little further or choose smaller size tracheostomy tube. Application of too much pressure while introducing the tracheostomy tube may cause inversion of adjoining tracheal rings inside the tracheal lumen which may work as a nidus for tracheal stenosis. Some times a little twisting motion and generous lubrication may help in passing the tube. The inserted tracheostomy tube should not be too long or too short. A small tube is vulnerable for inadvertent decannulation while longer tube may rub the carina and make the patient uncomfortable. If it is so, the tracheostomy tube must be changed with appropriate size and length.

Monitoring

There are no published guidelines for monitoring during formation of percutaneous dilational tracheostomy. As there is risk of dislodgement of airway device[24], hypoventilation, cardiac arrhythmias, entrapment of air in lungs due to occupation of tracheal lumen with the dilator [25,26] during formation of tracheal stoma, the author recommends a minimum of followings: Continuous monitoring of EKG, blood pressure, Oxygen saturation (SpO_2), end tidal carbon dioxide ($EtCO_2$) and peak airway pressure (PAP). The inspired oxygen concentration should be kept at 100% and the efforts must be made to maintain $SpO_2 > 95\%$ and $EtCO_2 < 50$ mm.Hg during the procedure. It is desirable to perform the percutaneous tracheostomy (at least first 10) under bronchoscopic (fiberoptic or rigid) control where the operator can visualize the tracheal puncture needle in the midline, guide wire and insertion of the dilators in tracheal lumen.[27,28]

There have been reports of paratracheal placement of tracheostomy tube. Following placement of tracheostomy tube its correct position in trachea must be verified. Monitoring of oxygen saturation is not a very reliable test of misplacement of tube as patient who breathed 100% oxygen and have good lung function may take several minutes to desaturate. Suction catheter may pass down in a false track and auscultation of chest may also give false impression of tracheostomy tube in trachea. A list of various tests and their reliability to confirm correct placement of tracheal tube are mentioned in Table 12.1. Bronchoscopic visualization of tracheal rings and carina through the tracheostomy tube is the most reliable method. This also enables the operator to look inside for tracheal injuries.

Table 12.1: Methods of verification of tube placement in the trachea

Absolutely reliable:
- Fiberoptic bronchoscopic visualization of tracheal rings/carina through the tube

Very reliable:
- $EtCO_2$ (but not in case of no cardiac output)
- Esophageal detector device

Reliable: (use multiple methods)
- Inflation of chest
- Auscultation of chest and epigastrium
- Condensation of moisture in ETT during expiration
- Sustained maintenance of SpO_2
- Passage of suction catheter
- Airway pressure

At the end of the procedure manual examination of chest and neck should be performed to diagnose appearance of surgical emphysema, if any. The chest should be inspected and auscultated to verify bilateral air entry into the lungs and to rule out development of pneumothorax.

In the initial years of introduction of percutaneous tracheostomy techniques in clinical practice bronchoscopic guidance was not suggested as a necessary part of the procedure. Bronchoscopy may provide certain benefits, such as confirmation of needle placement, dilatation of stoma, and tracheostomy tube placement which may be quite useful during initial period of starting the procedure. Therefore, the general use of bronchoscope is recommended. However, several reports on the use of bronchoscope have raised concern about potential untoward side effects; such as increase in pCO_2 leading to measurable increase in intracranial pressure.[29,30] Prolonged broncho-scopy can lead to derecruitment of alveoli and decrease in pO_2 in susceptible patients; and is not known to decrease the complications such as pneumothorax.

Securing the Tracheostomy Tube

Various types of tracheostomy tube securing tapes are available that can be tied around the neck in neutral position. A sterile dressing must be kept around the stoma before tying the knot. It is important to check that the securing tape of tracheostomy tube around the neck is not too tight or too loose and that can be checked by inserting two fingers (Fig. 12.6) between the neck and ties. The knot of the securing tape should be made on the opposite side of internal jugular vein catheter, if present, so that a better hygiene can be maintained. Some operators fix the tube with surgical sutures to avoid inadvertent decannulation in first 72 hours

as reinsertion of tracheostomy tube in per-cutaneously formed tracheal stoma is very difficult. However, suturing may make dressing changes more difficult.

Post-tracheostomy Chest X-ray

A post-procedure chest X-ray is routinely requested. Chest X-ray not only helps in identifying the development of pneumothorax or surgical emphysema following tracheostomy but also provides us an objective evidence for the documentation in the era of increased medico-legal cases. Though the practice of routine chest X-ray following uncomplicated tracheostomy has been questioned,[31,32] most workers continue to have one. In authors view most ICU patients do require daily or alternate day chest X-ray then what is a big harm by having one after the tracheostomy.

At the end of the procedure a detailed note should be written in the case sheet describing the anesthesia techniques, method of PDT and type of tracheostomy tube used. Any untoward incident or complication encountered should also be documented. Personal experience and expertise are individualized, but also influenced to some greater or lesser extent by the institutional environments and culture.[33] Regarding the practice of percutaneous tracheostomy, most practitioners develop, with training and with experience, patterns of practice at their institute. This indicates that the best practice may not be, and should not always be, identical from institute to institute. Therefore, the interested clinicians should maintain their own data bank of such procedures for the record, periodic audit and evidence based change in practice, if necessary. A copy of audit sheet, (Appendix shows an audit sheet filled at our institute), is maintained for a long-term follow-up and three monthly audits.

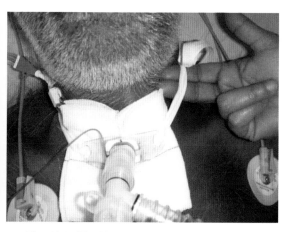

Fig. 12.6: Checking the ties of tracheostomy tube

APPENDIX

Audit proforma filled for all percutaneous tracheostomies at Sanjay Gandhi Postgraduate Institute of Medical Sciences, Lucknow (India)

Patient's Name   Age/Sex   CR No.

Diagnosis with relevant medical history in brief

Days on endotracheal tube/ventilator prior to tracheostomy

Indication for tracheostomy:

- Anticipating prolonged intubation or ventilation
- Slow weaning
- Failed extubation
- Others

Hemodynamic parameters before tracheostomy

- HR
- ABP
- CVP
- Any other

Respiratory parameters before tracheostomy (Mode of ventilation, FiO_2, level of PEEP, PAP, ABG, others)

Coagulation profile before tracheostomy:

- INR
- APTT
- Platelets

Anesthesia technique used: (GA/ Local + sedation)

Percutaneous tracheostomy kit used:

- Ciaglia (multiple dilators/Blue Rhino)
- Griggs' guidewire dilating forceps
- Frova's PercuTwist
- Ambesh T-Trach
- Fantoni's Translaryngeal tracheostomy
- Dolphin Balloon

Tracheostomy tube/size used

- Portex (blue line)
- Portex Bivona
- Rusch
- Shiley (non-fenestrated)

Guidance equipment used during tracheostomy:

- Fiberoptic bronchoscope
- Ultrasound (Preoperative scan/intraoperative)
- Both/none

Intraoperative complications/difficulties (if any):

Postoperative radiograph (findings):

Postoperative complications (if any):

Days (and date) of tracheostomy decannulation:

REFERENCES

1. Powell DM, Price PD, Forrest LA. Review of percutaneous tracheostomy. Laryngoscope 1998; 108:170-77.

2. Zgoda MA, Berger R. Balloon-facilitated percutaneous dilational tracheostomy tube placement: Preliminary report of a novel technique. Chest 2005;128:3688-90.

3. Shlugman D, Satya-Krishna R, Loh L. Acute fatal hemorrhage during percutaneous dilatational tracheostomy. Br J Anaesth 2003;90:517-20.

4. Schwann NM. Percutaneous dilational tracheostomy: Anesthetic consideration for a growing trend. Anesth Analg 1997;84:907-11.

5. Day C, Rankin N. Laceration of the cuff of an endotracheal tube during percutaneous dilational tracheostomy. Chest 1994;105:644.

6. Williams P, Warwick R. Gray's anatomy, 36th edn. London; Churchill Livingstone, 1980;1229.

7. Luntely JB, Kirkpatrick T. Tracheal tube placement during percutaneous dilational tracheostomy. Anaesthesia 1994;49:736.

8. Ambesh SP, Singh DK, Bose N. Use of a bougie to prevent accidental dislodgment of endotracheal tube during bedside percutaneous dilatational tracheostomy. Anesth Analg 2001;93:1364-5.

9. Tarpy JJ, Lynch L. The use of laryngeal mask airway to facilitate the insertion of a percutaneous tracheostomy. Intens Care Med 1994;20:448-9.

10. Dosemeci L, Yilmaz M, Gurpinar F, Ramazanoglu A. The use of laryngeal mask airway as an alternative to the endotracheal tube during percutaneous dilatational tracheostomy. Intens Care Med 2002;28:63-7.

11. Craven RM, Laver SR, Cook TM, Nolan JP. Use of the pro-seal LMA facilitates percutaneous dilatational tracheostomy. Can J Anaesth 2003;50:718-20.

12. Linstedt U, Moller F, Grote N, Zenz M, Prengel A. Intubating laryngeal mask as a ventilatory device during percutaneous dilatational tracheostomy: A descriptive study. Br J Anaesth 2007;99:912-5.

13. Treu TM, Knoch M, Focke N, Schulz M. Die perkutane dilatative tracheotomie als neues verfahren in der intensivmedizin. Durchfuhrung, Vorteile und Risiken. Dtsch Med Wochenschr 1997;122:599-605.

14. Ambesh SP, Sinha PK, Tripathi M, Matreja P. Comparison of laryngeal mask airway versus endotracheal tube ventilation to facilitate bedside percutaneous tracheostomy: A prospective comparative study. J Postgrad Med 2002;46:11-5.

15. Grundling M, Kuhn SO, Riedel T, Feyerherd F, Wendt M. Application of laryngeal mask for elective percutaneous dilatational tracheotomy. Anaethesiol Reanimat 1998;23:32-6.

16. Girgin NK, Kahveci SF, Yavascaoglu B, Kutlay O. A comparison of laryngeal mask airway and cuffed oropharyngeal airway during percutaneous tracheostomy. Saudi Med J 2007;28:1139-41.

17. Kaya FN, Gergin NK, Yavascaoglu B, Kahveci F, Korfali G. The use of laryngeal mask airway and the cuffed oropharyngeal airway during percutaneous tracheostomy. Ulus Travma Acil Cerrahi Derg 2006;12:282-7.

18. Roberts L, Cockroft S. Combitube and percutaneous tracheostomy. Anaesthesia 1998;53:716.

19. Letheren MJ, Parry N, Slater RM. A complication of percutaneous tracheostomy whilst using the combitube for airway control. Eu J Anaesthesiol 1997;14:464-6.

20. Mallick A, Quinn AC, Bodenham AR, Vucevic M. Use of the combitube for airway maintenance during percutaneous dilatational tracheostomy. Anaesthesia 1998;53:249-55.

21. Hartfield A, Bodenham A. Portable ultrasonic scanning of the anterior neck before percutaneous dilatational tracheostomy. Anaesthesia 1999;54:660-3.

22. Sustic A, Kovac D, Zgaljardic Z, Zupan Z, Krstulovic B. Ultrasound-guided percutaneous dilatational tracheostomy: A safe method to avoid cranial misplacement of the tracheostomy tube. Intensive Care Med 2000;26:1379-81.

23. Williams PL (ed.) Gray's Anatomy, 38th Edn. London: Churchill Livingstone, 1995:1530.

24. Freidman Y, Mayer AD. Bedside percutaneous tracheostomy in critically ill patients. Chest 1993;104: 532-5.

25. Ambesh SP, Pandey CK, Srivastava S, Agarwal A, Singh DK. Percutaneous tracheostomy with single dilatation technique: A prospective, randomized comparison of Ciaglia blue rhino versus Griggs guide wire dilating forceps. Anesth Analg 2002;95:1739-45.

26. Ambesh SP, Kaushik S. Percutaneous dilational tracheostomy: The Ciaglia method vs the Portex method. Anesth Analg 1998;87:556-61.

27. Barba CA, Angood PB, Kaudar DR, et al. Bronchoscopic guidance makes percutaneous tracheostomy a safe, cost effective, and easy to teach procedure. Surgery 1995; 118:879-83.

28. Winkler WB, Karnick R, Seelmann O. Bedside percutaneous dilational tracheostomy with endoscopic guidance: Experience with 71 ICU patients. Intens Care Med 1994;20:476-9.

29. Reilly PM, Anderson 3rd HL, Sing RF, Schwab CW, Barlett RH. Occult hypercarbia. An unrecognized phenomenon during percutaneous endoscopic tracheostomy. Chest 1995;107:1760-3.

30. Ernst A, Critchlow J. Percutaneous tracheostomy - special considerations. Clin Chest Med 2003;24: 409-12.

31. Tyroch AH. Routine chest radiograph is not indicated after open tracheostomy. Am Surg 2002;68:80-2.

32. Datta D. Utility of chest radiographs following percutaneous tracheostomy. Chest 2003;123:1603-6

33. Littlewood KE. Evidence base management of tracheostomies in hospitalized patients. Respir Care 2005; 50:516-8.

Chapter 13

Complications and Contraindications of Percutaneous Tracheostomy

Sushil P Ambesh

The decision to place tracheostomy should be made by considering the balance between benefits versus risks of potential complications. Further, it is very important to weigh advantages and disadvantages of percutaneous vs surgical tracheostomy on the basis of anatomical and pathophysiological factors of the patient. Though, most of the risks and benefits are not precisely known for any particular surgical technique and in most clinical situations, best understood factors must be taken in account. In general more difficult patients are usually subjected for open surgical tracheostomy rather than percutaneous tracheostomy. While in decision making with any technical procedure the level of experience of the operator will influence the outcome and risk.

Tracheostomy may be associated with numerous intraoperative and postoperative complications. A number of clinically important unique late complications have been recognized as well. The clinical relevance of these complications is considerable. Tracheostomy complications are traditionally categorized as early (occurring intraoperatively or within 24 hours), intermediate (occurring between 24 hours to one month period) and late (that occurs after a month to years together)

(Table 13.1). During the first week after tracheostomy, a mature tracheocutaneous track may not be developed. Inadvertent decannulation with efforts to reinsert the tracheostomy tube can result in misplacement into pretracheal fascia, leading to upper airway obstruction and asphyxia.[1] In such situations trachea should be re-intubated orally to provide immediate airway control and reinsertion of the tracheostomy tube may be done electively.

HEMORRHAGE

Unlike surgical tracheostomy, the technique of percutaneous tracheostomy does not provide controlled hemostasis and therefore bleeding is one of the complications. Although significant bleeding during PDT occurs infrequently,[2,3] bleeding complications from PDT from pretracheal vascular structures could be fatal.[4] A number of case reports of fatalities secondary to massive hemorrhage related to PDT include bleeding from pretracheal veins and arteries.[5,6] The bleeding could be from anterior blood vessels of neck or inside from tracheal mucosa lacerations. Minor bleeding varying from oozing requiring dressing changes to bleeding requiring only digital pressure to control, occurred in 20% of cases.[7,8] In most cases, bleeding usually

Table 13.1: Complications of tracheostomy

Early
- Hypoxemia
- Cardiac dysrrhythmias, hypotension
- Bronchospasm
- Hemorrhage
- Surgical trauma - esophagus, recurrent laryngeal nerve
- Pneumothorax, pneumomediastinum
- Subcutaneous emphysema
- Injury to neck vessels
- Misplacement of tracheostomy tube
- Inadvertent decannulation
- Tracheal ring rupture and herniation
- Posterior tracheal wall perforation
- Cardiac arrest, death

Intermediate
- Stoma site infection
- Tracheal erosion
- Tube displacement
- Tube obstruction
- Subcutaneous emphysema
- Tracheoesophageal fistula
- Aspiration and lung abscess

Late
- Tracheoesophageal fistula (TOF)
- Tracheoinnominate artery fistula (TIF)
- Persistent tracheocutaneous fistula
- Tracheal grannulomas
- Tracheal stenosis
- Tracheal dilatation
- Tracheomalacia

stops with lateral pressure applied by the tracheostomy tube or with direct pressure applied to the lateral walls of the tracheal stoma. Major bleeding necessitating blood transfusion or surgical intervention occurred in fewer than 5% patients and was usually venous in origin.[7,9-13] In such situations, insertion of endotracheal tube and inflation of cuff at the site of tracheal stoma along with application of direct external pressure locally help in controlling the bleeding. If bleeding is still continued, surgical help may be necessary. Recently, aortic arch laceration with lethal hemorrhagic complication after percutaneous tracheostomy has been reported in a patient with aberrant vascular anatomy.[14] Ultrasound scanning of the pretracheal tissues for presence of blood vessels at the intended site of tracheostomy and nearby structures is very helpful and is described in Chapter 19 of this book.

Delayed hemorrhage may also occur due to secondary hemostatic defect particularly in patients with multiple organ failure, renal failure, hepatic failure or multiple trauma that can lead to a life threatening complication of airway obstruction.[15] An unusual case of 'ball valve' clot obstruction of tracheostomy tube has been reported.[16] The problem of tracheal clot may be diagnosed by bronchoscopy. If there is an acute airway obstruction, the best approach is to remove the tracheostomy tube immediately and intubate the trachea with an endotracheal tube.

Tracheal Mucosa and Cartilagenous Injury

During formation of PDT, the flexibility of the cartilage allows the anterior tracheal surface to be significantly displaced proximally and distally to the intended tracheostoma placement.[17] Injury probably occurs as pressure from the tracheostomy deforms the anterior tracheal wall, resulting in macroscopic and microscopic stress fractures of the surrounding cartilaginous rings. Pressure on a less distensible calcified trachea has a lower fracture threshold. Van Heurn et al, in an autopsy findings, showed 11 out of 12 patients had fractures of one or more cartilaginous rings, while two of whom had fractured cricoids.[18] Concomitant mucosal injury with cartilage injury in patients having undergone PDT probably initiates an intense inflammatory response that, together with retained tracheal secretions and potential cuff injury, may in part explain the pathophysiology of tracheal stenosis. Post-tracheostomy bronchoscopic examination of trachea is useful in diagnosing the injury. Most such injuries heal spontaneously however, the chances of granulation formation increase.

Perforation of Posterior Tracheal Wall

Among the few complications, perforation of the posterior tracheal wall is the complication feared most, and its incidence appears to vary widely from nearly zero to 12.5%.[19-21] With tracheal perforation, persistent air leakage from the trachea can cause pneumothorax, pneumomediastinum, and pneumopericardium, and therefore air leakage must be stopped immediately. Every tracheal perforation should require an esophagoscopy to exclude its perforation, and in doubtful situations, a chest CT scan. Tracheal injuries, independent of their origin, are life threatening incidents, and surgical repair has been recommended as the treatment of choice. Recommendation for surgical repair is based on the assumption that tracheal perforation otherwise results in mediastinitis or subsequent tracheal stenosis.[22] Beiderlinden et al encountered five patients of tracheal perforation, two in the trachea's upper-third and three in its middle-third following the PDT.[21] They bridged the tracheal defects conservatively by endotracheal or tracheostomy tubes under bronchoscopic guidance and the cuff was inflated distal to the lesion. Air leakage stopped immediately and all tracheal defects healed without further interventions. No case of mediastinitis or tracheal stenosis was observed.

For lesions below or close to carina and hemodynamic instability, emergency thoracotomy with surgical repair may be the treatment of choice. Persistent air leak despite positioning of the tracheal tube just above the carina also limits a conservative approach, indicating a defect too close to the bifurcation for the bridging. However, as long as the defect is localized in the trachea's upper or middle third, conservative treatment by bridging the defect by placing the artificial airway can be performed quickly with no additional risk.

Misplacement of Tracheostomy Tube

Misplacement of tracheostomy tube into the paratracheal tissues, posterior tracheal wall, esophagus and intrapleural spaces[23] have all been reported with percutaneous tracheostomy insertion. However, the incidence varies with type of PDT techniques used and the experience of the operator. Therefore, correct placement of tracheostomy tube must be ensured by bilateral air entry into the chest, monitoring of $EtCO_2$ and direct visualization of tracheal tube in the trachea.

Pneumothorax/surgical Emphysema

A number of cases of subcutaneous emphysema, mediastinal emphysema, pneumothorax and pneumomediastinum (Fig. 13.1) have been reported in the literature;[24] however, the incidence (<1%) are not worrisome. After formation of PDT, the neck, supraclavicular and infraclavicular area of the patient must be palpated for presence of surgical emphysema; and bilateral air entry into the chest must be ascertained by auscultation. Monitoring of airway pressure, SpO_2 and $EtCO_2$ are essential. We advocate that all patients must have chest radiographs after PDT, though not all workers agree, to exclude development of pneumothorax or other barotrauma. If there is evidence of pneumothorax, intercostal water seal drainage must be instituted without delay.

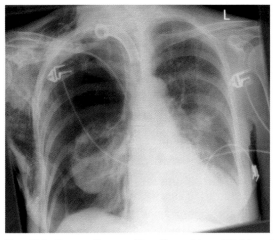

Fig. 13.1: Pneumothorax with collapsed lung (Right) and surgical emphysema following percutaneous dilational trachesotomy with Ciaglia's Blue Rhino

Tracheal Stenosis

The average internal diameter of an adult trachea is 2.5 cm, and the subglottic space that is defined as the area 5 mm below the vocal cords to the under surface of the cricoid cartilage has an average internal diameter of 1.7 cm. The most crucial long-term complication of tracheostomy is tracheal stenosis.[25] It is an abnormal narrowing of the tracheal lumen, most commonly occurs at the level of the stoma or above the stoma but below the vocal cords. Tracheal stenosis may also occur at the site of tracheostomy tube cuff or at the site of the tube's tip. Tracheal stenosis following tracheostomy, irrespective of the methods used, can occur at microscopic and macroscopic levels. Microscopic stenosis occurs in almost all cases. However, clinically significant macroscopic stenosis occurs when the tracheal diameter is reduced to <50% of its original diameter.[26,27] Norwood et al reported 31% incidence of 10% tracheal stenosis on computed tomography and 2% had severe stenosis reducing tracheal lumen to more than 50%.[28] All these stenosis were seen at the site of tracheal stoma, with no stenosis at the level of cannula tip or cuff. Hotchkiss et al reported two cases of severe tracheal stenosis (70% tracheal lumen occlusion) following decannulation of percutaneous tracheostomy where one patient had to undergo anterior wedge resection and cartilaginous graft.[29] Stomal stenosis develops secondary to bacterial infection and chondritis that weaken the anterior and lateral tracheal walls. Multiple risk factors are associated with stomal stenosis, including sepsis, stomal infection, hypotension, advanced age, male sex, steroids, tight fitting or oversized cannula, excessive tube movement, prolonged placement and disproportionate excision of anterior tracheal cartilage during formation of the tracheostomy.

Suprasternal stenosis has recently been reported, particularly as a complication of PDT.[30-32] Investigations on the most commonly used PDT technique, the Ciaglia method, have reported varying degrees of tracheal stenosis.[33-37] Dollner et al,[38] have shown that the tracheal stenosis in patients with Griggs' technique is similar and comparable with Ciaglia's technique. Several theories relating to causes of tracheal stenosis after PDT have been proposed in the literature, including aberrant placement of the tracheostomy and increased insertional pressure on the cartilage. Involvement of the cricoid cartilage (with triangular angulation) and fracture of first tracheal ring (gothic arch deformation) has been shown as one of the predisposing factor of tracheal stenosis.[38,39] The characteristic feature of this kind of stenosis is caving-in of the anterior tracheal wall by the fractures protruding into the tracheal lumen.

Other location of tracheal stenosis is at the site of tracheal cuff (infrastomal) due to ischemic injury to the tracheal mucosa. This occurs when cuff pressure exceeds the perfusion pressure of the capillaries of the tracheal wall. Shearing forces from the tube or the cuff may further aggravate injury to the airway. The incidence of infrastomal stenosis has fallen 10-fold with the introduction of high volume low pressure cuffs.[40-41] Unfortunately, overinflation of high-volume low-pressure cuff also can lead to ischemic airway injury. With prolonged ischemia, mucosal ulceration, chondritis, and cartilaginous necrosis may ensue, leading to formation of granulation tissue and tracheal stenosis.

Another site of tracheal stenosis is near the distal tip of the tracheal tube. Depending on the positioning of the tube, the tip may rub against either the anterior or the posterior tracheal wall. This may lead to injury to the posterior tracheal wall resulting into stenosis or tracheoesophageal fistula.

Therefore, all patients who had undergone PDT must be followed to look for tracheal stenosis. The clinician should have high index of suspicion in patients who can not be weaned from mechanical ventilation or who can not be decannulated. Alternatively, tracheal stenosis may present as unexplained dyspnea weeks to months after decannulation. Though there is no definite time interval, however, it is prudent to follow these patients for at least 3 months to 2 years.

It is very important to remember that tracheal stenosis may be asymptomatic until the lumen has been reduced by 50-70%. The initial manifestations may be increased cough and difficulty in clearing secretions. Once the tracheal lumen is reduced to < 10 mm, exertional dyspnea occurs. When the lumen is narrowed to < 5 mm, dyspnea at rest or stridor is seen. The patient should be subjected to a battery of investigations for imaging of the tracheal air column that include chest radiography, tracheal tomography, CT and magnetic resonance imaging. Laryngotracheoscopy or bronchoscopy is important to define the exact site of stenosis, the cause of stenosis and length of stenosed segment.

In symptomatic patients the neodymium-Yttrium-aluminium-garnet (Nd-YAG) laser excision with or without rigid bronchoscopic dilation is the most preferred approach. Suprasternal granulation tissue can be excised by sharp dissection under bronchoscopic guidance. In patients where laser resection is not possible, stenting of the airway or surgical repair are the next best options. The most effective treatment of tracheal stenosis is tracheal resection and primary anastomosis.[42,43] However, the surgery for tracheal stenosis in the subglottic region could be complex because two important nerves, the recurrent laryngeal nerve and external branch of superior laryngeal nerve, lie in the close proximity.

Tracheoinnominate Artery Fistula

The TIF is a rare but one of the most feared complication with an estimated incidence of 0.1-1%.[44,45] Initial case reports of TIF resulted from surgically performed tracheostomies. However, the incidence may have declined because of advances in tracheostomy tube technology, introduction of PDT and post-tracheostomy care. It results in a high mortality, even in cases where successful initial surgical repair was accomplished.[45] Therefore, we suggest that TIF, though rare, should be borne in mind by all those involved in tracheostomy management. Pressure necrosis from high cuff pressure, mucosal erosion from malpositioned tracheostomy tube, tracheal incision, excessive neck movement, dragging of ventilator tube, radiotherapy or prolonged intubation have all been implicated in TIF formation. A high lying innominate artery, particularly in thin built or poorly nourished patient, may act as a risk factor in TIF formation. Several authors suggest that a low lying tracheostomy tube is an obvious cause of fistula formation.[46] However, even when the tracheostomy is placed between second and third tracheal rings, as recommended, these complications can still occur. The best preventive and treatment strategies are to avoid placing PDT below the 4th tracheal ring, avoiding hyperextension of the neck, use of high-volume low-pressure cuff cannula (cuff pressure < 20 mm Hg) and early suspicion of presence of TIF.[47]

Any peristomal bleed or hemostasis should warn to initiate full clinical investigation for the underlying cause. Hemorrhage within 48 hours of tracheostomy is typically associated with local tissue vessel trauma (anterior jugular or inferior thyroid veins), systemic coagulopathy, tracheal mucosa erosion secondary to tracheal suction or bronchopneumonia. Vascular erosion from a tracheostomy tube leading to formation of TIF requires longer time, generally more than a week. Occurrence of hemorrhage from tracheostomy between one to six week period should give rise a suspicion of TIF until proven otherwise.[48] A sentinel bleed is reported in more than 50% of patients who then develop massive delayed haemorrhage.[46,49,50] Rarely, hemorrhage occurring after six weeks is related to TIF and in such cases most likely cause could be granulation tissue, tracheobronchitis or malignancy.

Management of a suspected TIF will depend upon whether there is active bleeding into the airway hindering adequate ventilation. Immediate bronchoscopy is advocated to visualize the site and extent of bleeding however, it may not be feasible in severe active bleeding. Overinflation of the tracheal tube cuff may provide airway protection and may control the bleeding temporarily. If, however, bleeding continues then pressure dressing should be applied to the stoma site that may temporarily control bleeding by direct temponade effect in more than 80% of patients.[51] As long as airway remains free of blood; no attempt should be made to manipulate the tracheostomy tube. The patient should be shifted in operation room for surgical exploration and repair of TIF without delay. Mortality is 100% without operative intervention.

Tracheoesophageal Fistula

Tracheoesophageal fistula, a connection between trachea and esophagus, is an uncommon but serious and often fatal complication, occurring in less than 1% of patients on prolonged tracheostomy.[52] It may be iatrogenic resulting from injury to the posterior tracheal wall during formation of percutaneous dilatational tracheostomy. Alternatively, longstanding high cuff pressure or the tip of the tracheostomy tube can cause posterior tracheal wall erosion and subsequently fistula formation.[53] The presence of nasogastric tube, and resulting esophageal injury, may facilitate development of this life threatening complication.[54,55] Tracheoesophageal fistula as well as tracheoinnominate artery fistula together has been reported in a patient who had tracheostomy for four months.[56] Tracheoesophageal fistula may manifest as the copious production of secretions and recurrent aspiration of food. On suctioning through endotracheal tube, food material may be noticed. Water dye given by mouth may be traced into the trachea on bronchoscopy. Generally, these patients develop severe gastric distension due to

movement of respiratory air into the stomach via fistula. Barium esophagography and CT scan of the mediastinum are helpful in diagnosing the fistula. Treatment includes placement of tracheal as well as esophageal stent (double stenting). In patients who are capable of tolerating the thoracic surgery may be considered for surgical repair.

Tracheomalacia/ Tracheal Dilatation

Localized pressure exerted by the inflatable cuff of endotracheal or tracheostomy tubes on the tracheal wall can rarely cause reversible or persistent tracheal dilatation, depending on the duration of the tube.[57] This comprises a potentially life-threatening situation by means of tracheal rupture,[58] ventilation failure,[59] aspiration and secondary stenosis at the same level or tracheal collapse on forced expiration after weaning from ventilator.[60] The capillary perfusion pressure of the tracheal mucosa is 25-30 mm Hg and a lower cuff pressure is required to prevent ischemia necrosis. Contributing factors are hypoxemia, sepsis, steroids and hypotension.[61] Less commonly, additional ulceration, softening and fragmentation of the tracheal cartilage leads to tracheomalacia that may manifest as dilatation. Tracheal dilatation should be suspected when increasing volumes of air are required for adequate cuff seal. The complication may be diagnosed as an incidental finding on a chest X-ray (Fig. 13.2), CT scan or flexible bronchoscopy.

The management of tracheal dilatation is difficult and most reports emphasize the importance of prevention or avoidance of progression of the complication.[62,63] Important factors are aseptic tracheal suction, aseptic tube replacement and inflation pressure less than 20 mm Hg. Periodic deflation of the balloon is of little help in preventing trcacheomalacia.[59] The methods suggested to prevent tracheal dilatation are use of tracheal tubes with two cuffs (Fig. 13.3), inflated alternately[64] or periodic change of tracheal cuff position by altering

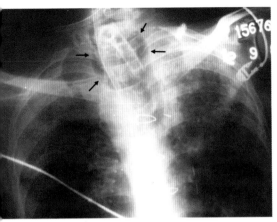

Fig. 13.2: Tracheal dilatation (marked with arrows) in a tracheostomized patient of malignant myasthenic syndrome who remained on ventilator for about 11 months

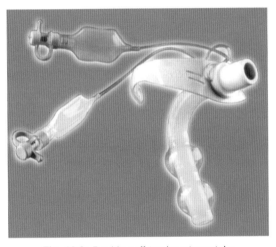

Fig. 13.3: Double cuff tracheostomy tube
(SIMS Portex, UK)

the length of tube with the help of adjustable flange.[65] Other method that can be justifiable is the use of automated cuff pressure that prevents arbitrary manual overinflation.[66]

Contraindications of percutaneous tracheostomy

What constitutes absolute and relative contraindications for percutaneous tracheostomy has become a matter of debate. Most published articles consider cervical injury, pediatric age, coagulopathy, and emergency airway necessity as absolute contraindications, whereas short, fat neck and obesity are relative contraindications. However, several reports have recently emerged suggesting safety and feasibility of performing PCT in patients with the previously described contraindications.[67-72]

A retrospective study by Blankenship[68] suggests percutaneous tracheostomy may be performed safely in the morbidly obese patient as long as anterior neck landmarks can be palpated and in the coagulopathic patient with platelets as low as 17,000 and International Normalized Ratio >1.5. Tabaee et al[72] demonstrated the safety of PDT in patients with short neck lengths in their prospective, randomized study. The PDT was found to be safe and feasible even in emergency trauma cases in a case series study by Ben-Nun (2004).[67] In a restrospective study Gravvanis et al [70] showed that PDT can be safely and more rapidly performed in burned patients with associated inhalation injury at the bedside. Percutaneous tracheostomy was also found to be safe and feasible in patients with cervical spine fractures in a case series by Ben-Nun et al (2006).[71]

At present absolute contraindications, though may change later, are as follows:
- Patient age younger than 10 years
- Necessity of emergency airway access because of acute airway compromise
- Gross distortion of the neck anatomy due to the following:
  - Hematoma
  - Tumor
  - Thyromegaly (second or third degree)
  - High innominate artery
  - Contracture neck

The relative contraindications are as follows:
- Patient obesity with short neck that obscures neck landmarks

- Medically uncorrectable bleeding diatheses
  - Prothrombin time or activated partial thromboplastin time more than 1.5 times the reference range
  - Platelet count less than 50,000/μL
- Bleeding time longer than 10 minutes
- Need for positive end-expiratory pressure (PEEP) of more than 20 cm of water
- Evidence of infection in the soft tissues of the neck at the prospective surgical site.

REFERENCES

1. Reibel JF. Tracheostomy/tracheotomy. Respir Care 1999;44:820-23.
2. Freeman BD, Isabella K, Cobb JP, et al. A prospective randomized study comparing percutaneous with surgical tracheostomy in critically ill patients. Crit Care Med 2001;29:926-30.
3. Al-Ansari MA, Hijari MH. Clinical review: Percutaneous dilational tracheostomy. Crit Care 2006;10:202.
4. Shlugman D, Satya-Krishna R, Loh L. Acute fatal haemorrhage during percutaneous dilatational tracheostomy. Br J Anaesth 2003;90:517-20.
5. McCormick B, Manara AR. Mortality from percutaneous dilatational tracheostomy. A report of three cases. Anaesthesia 2005;60:490-5.
6. Kearney PA, Griffen MM, Ochoa JB, et al. A single centre 8-yr experience with percutaneous dilational tracheostomy. Ann Surg 2000;231:701-9.
7. Crofts SL, Alzeer A, McGuire GP, et al. A comparison of percutaneous and operative tracheostomies in intensive care patients. Can J Anaesth 1995;42:775-9.
8. Holdgaard HO, Pedersen J, Jensen RH, et al. Percutaneous dilatational tracheostomy versus conventional surgical tracheostomy. Acta Anaesthesiol Scand 1998;42:545-50.
9. Muhammad JK, Major E, Wood a, et al. Percutaneous dilatational tracheostomy: Haemorrhagic complications and the vascular anatomy of the anterior neck. A review base on 497 cases. Int J Oral Maxillofac Surg 2000;29:217-22.
10. Hazard P, Jones C, Benitone J. Comparative clinical trials of standard operative tracheostomy with percutaneous tracheostomy. Crit Care Med 1991; 19:1018-24.
11. Friedman Y, Fildes J, Mizock B, et al. Comparison of percutaneous and surgical tracheostomies. Chest 1996;110:480-5.
12. VanHeurn LWE, VanGeffen GJ, Brink PRG. Clinical experience with percutaneous dilatational tracheostomy. Eur J Surg 1996;162:531-5.
13. Porter JM, Ivatury RR. Preferred route of tracheostomy-percutaneous versus open at the bedside: A randomized prospective study in the surgical intensive care unit. Am Surg 1999;65:142-6.
14. Ayoub OM, Griffiths MV. Aortic arch laceration: A lethal complication after percutaneous tracheostomy. Laryngoscope 2007;117:176-8.
15. Bernard SA, Jones BM, Shearer WA. Percutaneous dilatational tracheostomy complicated by delayed life-threatening haemorrhage. Aust N Z J Surg 1992;62: 152-3.
16. Skowronski GA, Bersten AD, Vedig AE. Bleeding risk with percutaneous tracheostomy. Intens Care Med 1990;18:273.
17. Kearney PA, Griffen MM, Ochoa JB, Boulanger BR, Tseui BJ, Mentzer RM. A single center 8-year experience with percutaneous dilational tracheostomy. Ann Surg 2000;231:701-9.
18. Van Heurn LW, Theunissen PH, Ramsay G, Brink PR. Pathophysiologic changes of the trachea after percutaneous dilational tracheostomy. Chest 1996;109466-9.
19. Beiderlinden M, Aalz MK, sander A, et al. Complications of bronchoscopically guided percutaneous dilational tracheostomy: Beyond the learning curve. Intensive Care Med 2002;28:59-62.
20. Trottier SJ, Hazard PB, Sakabu SA, et al. Posterior tracheal wall perforation during percutaneous dilational tracheostomy. Chest 1999;115:1383-9.
21. Beiderlinden M, Adamzik M, Peters J. Conservative treatment of tracheal injuries. Anesth Analg 2005;100:210-4.
22. Weissberg D, Utkin V. Airway trauma: Tracheobronchial trauma. In: Webb WR, Besson A (Eds). Thoracic Surgery: Surgical management of chest injuries. St. Louis: Mosby Year Book, 1991:392-6.
23. Noden JB, Kirkpatrick T. Intrapleural percutaneous tracheostomy. Anaesthesia 1995;50:91.
24. Matsuura K, Nakanisi T, Nagakawa T, Katou S, Honda Y. Massive subcutaneous emphysema following percutaneous tracheostomy. Masui 2008;57:474-8.
25. McFarlane C, Denholm SW, Sudlow CLM, et al. Laryngotracheal stenosis: A serious complication of percutaneous tracheostomy. Anaesthesia 1994;49: 38-40.
26. Streitz JM, Shapshay SM. Airway injury after tracheostomy and endotracheal intubation. Surg Clin North Am 1991;71:1211-30.

27. Finucane BT, Santora AH. Anatomy of the airway. In: Finucane BT, Santora AH, (Eds). Principles of airway management. 2nd edn. Boston MA: Mosby, 1996;1-18.
28. Norwood S, Vallina VL, Short K, Saigusa M, Fernandez LG, McLarty JW. Incidence of tracheal stenosis and other late complications after percutaneous tracheostomy. Ann Surg 2000;232:233-41.
29. Hotchkiss KS, McCaffrey JC. Laryngotracheal injury after percutaneous dilational tracheostomy in cadaver specimens. Laryngoscope 2003;113:16-20.
30. Benjamin B, Kertesz T. Obstructive suprasternal granulation tissue following percutaneous tracheostomy. Anaesth Intensive Care 1999;27:596-600.
31. Brichet A, Verkindre C, Dupont J, Carlier ML, Darras J, Wurtz A, et al. Multidisciplinary approach to management of post intubation tracheal stenoses. Eur Resp J 1999;13:888-93.
32. Koitschev A, Graumueller S, Zenner HP, Dommerich S, Simon C. Tracheal stenosis and obliteration above the tracheostoma after percutaneous dilational tracheostomy. Crit Care Med 2003;31:1574-6.
33. Walz MK, Peitgen K, Thurauf N, et al. Percutaneous dilatational tracheostomy: Early results and long-term outcome of 326 critically ill patients. Intensive Care Med 1998;24:685-90.
34. Rosenbower TJ, Morris JA Jr, Eddy VA, et al. The long-term complications of percutaneous dilatational tracheostomy. Am Surg 1998;64:82-86.
35. Wagner F, Nasseri R, Laucke U, et al. Percutaneous dilatational tracheostomy: Results and long-term outcome of critically ill patients following cardiac surgery. Thorac Cardivasc Surg 1998;46:352-6.
36. Law RC, Carney AS, Manara AR. Long-term outcome after percutaneous dilational tracheostomy. Anaesthesia 1997;52:51-6.
37. Fischler MP, Kuhn M, Cantieni R, et al. Late outcome of percutaneous dilatational tracheostomy in intensive care patients. Intensive Care Med 1995;21:475-81.
38. Dollner R, Verch M, Schweiger P, Deluigi C, Graf B, Wallner F. Laryngotracheoscopic findings in long-term follow-up after Griggs tracheostomy. Chest 2002;122:206-12.
39. Raghuraman G, Rajan S, Marzouk JK, Mullhi D, Smith FG. Is tracheal stenosis caused by percutaneous tracheostomy different from that by surgical tracheostomy? Chest 2005;127:879-85.
40. Lewis FR Jr, Schiobohm RM, Thomas AN. Prevention of complications from prolonged tracheal intubation. Am J Surg 1978;135:452-7.
41. Leigh JM, Maynard JP. Pressure on the tracheal mucosa from cuffed tubes. BMJ 1979;1(6172):1173-4.
42. Fikkers BG, Briede IS, Verwiel JM, et al. Percutaneous tracheostomy with Blue Rhino technique: Presentation of 100 consecutive patients. Anaesthesia 2002;57:1094-7.
43. Donahue DM. Reoperative tracheal surgery. Chest Surg Clin N Am 2003;13:375-83.
44. Allan JS, Wright CD. Tracheoinnominate fistula: Diagnosis and management. Chest Surg Clin A Am 2003;13:331-41.
45. Grant CA, Dempsey G, Harrison J, Jones T. Tracheo-innominate artery fistula after percutaneous tracheostomy: Three case reports and a clinical review. Br J Anaesth 2006;96:127-31.
46. Grillo CG. Tracheal Fistula to Brachiocephalic Artery. In: Grillo CG, (Eds) Surgery of the Trachea and Bronchi. Hamilton: BC Decker, 2003; Ch. 13,1-9.
47. Ambesh SP, Kumar V, Srivastava K. Tracheo-innominate artery fistula. Anesth Analg 2000;90:231.
48. Nelems JM. Tracheo-innominate artery fistula. Am J Surg 1981;141:526-7.
49. Courcy PA, Rodriguez A, Garrett HE. Operative technique for repair of tracheoinnominate artery fistula. J Vasc Surg 1985;2:332-4.
50. Jones JW, Reynolds M, Hewitt RL, Drapanas T. Tracheoinnominate artery erosion: Successful surgical management of a devastating complication. Ann Surg 1976;184:194-204.
51. Bloss RS, Ward RE. Survival after tracheoinnominate artery fistula. Am J Surg 1980;139:251-3.
52. Reed MF, Mathisen DJ. Tracheoesophageal fistula. Chest Surg Clin North Am 2003;13:271-89.
53. Hameed AK, Mohamed H, Al-Mansoori M. Acquired tracheoesophageal fistula due to high intracuff pressure. Annals Thorac Med 2008;3:23-5.
54. Wood De, Mathisen DJ. Late complication of tracheostomy. Clin Chest Med 1991;12:597-609.
55. Dartevelle P, Macchiarini P. Management of acquired tracheoesophageal fistula. Chest Surg Clin North Am 1996;6:819-36.
56. Hung JJ, Hsu HS, Huang CS, Yang KY. Tracheoesophageal fistula and tracheo-subclavian artery fistula after tracheostomy. European J Cardiothoac Surg 2007;32:676-8.
57. Leverment JN, Pearson FG, Rae S. Tracheal size following tracheostomy with cuffed tracheostomy tubes: An experimental study. Thorax 1975;30:271-7.
58. Luna CM, Legarreta G, Esteva H, Laffaire E, Jolly EC. Effect of tracheal dilatation and rupture on mechanical ventilation using a low pressure cuff tube. Chest 1993;104:639-40.
59. Fryer ME, Marshall RD. Tracheal dilatation. Anaesthesia 1976;31:470-8.

60. Klausen N, Lomholt N, Qvist J. Dilatation of the trachea treated with NL-tracheostomy tube. Crit Care Med 1982;10:52-54.

61. Grillo HC, Cooper JD, Geffin B, Pontoppidan H. A low pressure cuff for tracheostomy tubes to minimize tracheal injury. J Thorac Cardiovasc Surg 1971;62:898-907.

62. Rhodes A, Lamb FJ, Grounds RM, Bennet ED. Tracheal dilatation complicating prolonged tracheal intubation. Anaesthesia 1997;52:70-2.

63. Kahn F, Reddy NC. Enlarging intratracheal tube cuff diameter: A quantitative roentgenographic study of its value in the early prediction of serious tracheal damage. Ann Thor Surg 1977;24:49-53.

64. Prinsley P. Ballooned trachea as a consequence of intubation. J Laryngol Otol 1992;106:561-2.

65. Cooper JD, Grillo HC. The evolution of tracheal injury due to ventilatory assistance through cuffed tubes: A pathologic study. Ann Surg 1969;169:334-48.

66. Lomholt N, Borgeskov S, Kirkby B. A new tracheostomy tube III: Bronchofibreoptic examination of the trachea after prolonged intubation with the NL tracheostomy tube. Acta Anaesth Scand 1981;25:407-11.

67. Ben-Nun A, Altman E, Best LA. Emergency percutaneous tracheostomy in trauma patients: An early experience. Ann Thorac Surg 2004;77:1045-7.

68. Blankenship DR, Kulbersh BD, Gourin CG, et al. High-risk tracheostomy: Exploring the limits of the percutaneous tracheostomy. Laryngoscope 2005; 115:987-9.

69. Kluge S, Meyer A, Kuhnelt P, et al. Percutaneous tracheostomy is safe in patients with severe thrombocytopenia. Chest 2004;126:547-51.

70. Gravvanis AI, Tsoutsos DA, Iconomou TG, et al. Percutaneous versus Conventional Tracheostomy in Burned Patients with Inhalation Injury. World J Surg 2005;29:1571-75.

71. BenNun A, Orlovsky M, Best LA. Percutaneous tracheostomy in patients with cervical spine fractures—feasible and safe. Interact Cardiovasc Thorac Surg 2006;5:427-9.

72. Tabaee A, Geng E, Lin J, Kakoullis S, McDonald B, Rodriguez H, et al. Impact of neck length on the safety of percutaneous and surgical tracheotomy: A prospective, randomized study. Laryngoscope 2005;115:1685-90.

Chapter 14

Percutaneous Dilational Tracheostomy in Special Situations

Sushil P Ambesh

INTRODUCTION

Tracheostomy is most often performed in critically ill patients as an elective procedure to provide airway access for prolonged mechanical ventilation, to assist weaning from ventilator, tracheobronchial toilet and relief of upper airway obstruction. Tracheostomy should not be a method of choice for the control of airway in patients with acute respiratory obstruction as it is associated with high complication rates; cricothyrotomy is the preferred procedure in this setting.[1] Tracheostomy can be performed by the standard open surgical technique or by percutaneous dilatational methods that do not require a surgical exposure of trachea. Since resurgence of interest in percutaneous dilatational tracheostomy (PDT), after Ciaglia's technique in 1985, more and more such procedures are being carried out in critically ill patients; however, it has been contraindicated in patients with morbid obesity, obscure cervical anatomy, short thick neck, active infection at the local site, previous tracheostomy, cervical spine fracture, burns, coagulation disorders and children below 12 years of age. Many of the suggested contraindications are not adequately supported with published data and are merely suggestions. Recent studies suggest that the PDT can be performed safely in obese patients,[2] previous tracheostomy[3] and many more

situations that are otherwise contraindicated with some modifications and precautions. It appears that the list of contraindications may decrease depending on the setting of the intensive care unit, type of kit used, bronchoscopic assistance and skill of the operators.

PDT IN SPECIAL SITUATIONS

Morbid Obesity

Morbidly obese patients admitted in ICU face a number of problems related to skin care, vascular access, nutrition, fluid management and also delay in shifting from translaryngeal intubation to tracheostomy. Due to their short, thick neck with obscure anatomical landmarks, these patients are included in the list of contraindications for PDT. However, the morbid obesity as the contraindication for PDT has never been supported by any trials. In a study, Mansharamani et al[2] performed PDT in 13 consecutive morbidly obese patients (BMI of 28-62) using a vertical incision and blunt dissection of pretracheal tissues. The vertical incision allowed the operator to feel and select the appropriate site for tracheal puncture without the need for reincision. Once the cricoid cartilage and tracheal rings were identifiable by palpation, the tracheal puncture needle was inserted, a guide wire placed and stoma dilated. All these patients were inserted with tracheostomy tube with extra-horizontal length. There were no complications or any particular technique difficulty and there were no failure in placement of planned tracheostomy tube. This study demonstrates that vertical skin incision and blunt dissection of subcutaneous fat greatly facilitates identification of tracheal landmarks. This experience has allowed us to perform PDT in morbidly obese patients (Fig. 14.1) without much time delay.

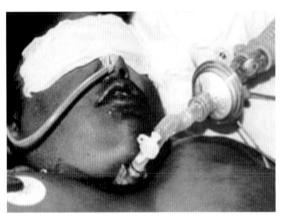

Fig. 14.1: Percutaneous dilatational tracheostomy with Ambesh "T-Trach" kit in a morbidly obese patient. Tracheostomy site is dressed with a povidine soaked gauze piece

Repeat Tracheostomy

The literature has frequently cited previous tracheostomy as one of the contraindications for the PDT[4,5] without any supporting clinical data. The author feels that these are precautionary measures especially for the learners. There are several case reports[6,7] and a study[3] that describe successful formation of PDT in patients who had had tracheostomy in the past. Meyer et al, in their 14 consecutive patients of repeat tracheostomy, used reincision of previous scar and insertion of needle through the tracheal defect, followed by dilatation and placement of tracheostomy tube of size 7 or 8 mm. They encountered no complications except an accidental late decannulation and judged the procedure as technically easy.

Emergency Percutaneous Tracheostomy

The requirement for an emergency airway had been considered to be an absolute contraindication to PDT; cricothyrotomy being the procedure of choice in this situation. In our opinion, this recommendation remains appropriate for those lacking experience. However, there have been several case reports (grade C evidence) of its safety and feasibility, in experienced hands, in emergency situations.[8-11] In one case endotracheal intubation past a retropharyngeal hematoma using a 5 mm tube provided inadequate oxygenation; this was improved by Ciaglia's PDT.[12] Dob et al have used the Portex technique in two cases to obviate the need for cricothyroidotomy, and to provide definite airway, without the risk of kinking.[13]

The author has performed a number of percutaneous tracheostomies using T-Trach kit in emergency situations to establish a definite airway; however, in all patients cricothyroidotomy cannula (14-gauze) was placed prior to performing the PDT (Figs 14.2A to D). In 17 cases of emergency PDT performed using T-Trach kit the author has not encountered any life threatening complications. All the procedures were done under local anesthesia. The procedure time has been between 3-5 minutes in all cases.

Children

PDT was originally considered to be contraindicated in children below 16 years of age. However, there have been number of case reports and series of PDTs successfully performed in children aged 5-16 years.[14,15] Zawadzka-Glos and Colleagues performed percutaneous tracheostomy in three children between 5 to 15 years of age using Fantoni's translaryngeal tracheostomy (TLT) technique under direct rigid bronchoscopy. The surgeries were performed in the near-drowned 5-year-old boy, and 15-year-old lupus erythematosus girl with a permanent brain damage resulted from a cardiac

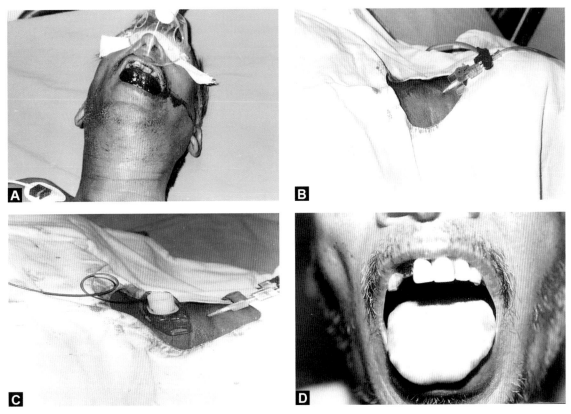

Figs 14.2A to D: (A) A patient of sublingual hematoma with severe upper airway obstruction. (B) 14-G cannula was inserted through cricothyroid membrane and oxygen administered. (C) Tracheostomy tube placed with T-Trach kit. (D) Same patient after a week at the time of discharge (bluish patches over the tongue are still visible).

arrest, 11-year-old cardiac girl with post-intubation laryngeal stenosis. In the first two cases, the procedure went uneventful; in one case the tube was accidentally pulled out during the rotation phase and surgical tracheostomy was performed. They concluded that TLT is especially suitable for children below 10 years of age and is associated with very few complications.[15] Fantoni and Ripamonti have reported successful formation of TLT in 14 children aged 2 months to 7 years.[16] The author has performed several PDTs in children between 5-10 years of age using Griggs' forceps with no significant complications (Fig. 14.3)

Cervical Spine Clearance

Cervical spine fracture is considered a relative contraindication to PDT due to inability to extend the neck. A complication rate of 7.1% has been reported in a case series of 28 patients who had undergone PDT without having cervical spine clearance.[17] Sustic et al, in another series of 16 patients with anterior cervical spine fusions following spinal cord injury had randomly assigned the patients either for surgical tracheostomy or ultrasound-guided PDT.[18] In terms of complications, US-guided PDT was as safe as surgical tracheostomy and was much quicker.

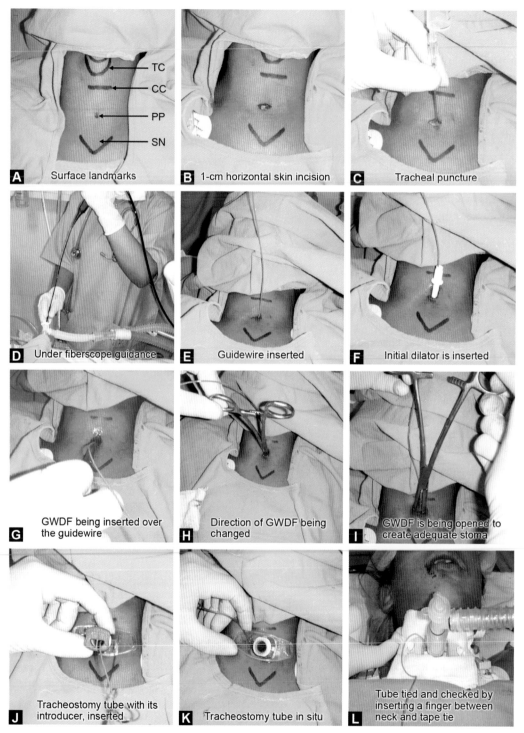

Fig. 14.3: Percutaneous tracheostomy in a 7-year old child with Griggs' guidewire dilating forceps

Severe Thrombocytopenia

Severe thrombocytopenia has been described as a contraindication to PDT. In a single centre, retrospective cohort study (Grade B evidence), Kluge et al[19] assessed the safety of PDT in ventilated patients with severe thrombocytopenia (platelets count <50,000/µL). They concluded that in the hands of experienced ICU staff, bronchoscopically guided PDT has a low complication rate; when platelets transfusions are given before the procedure; and when heparin therapy, even in those patients at very high risk for thromboembolic events, is interrupted during the procedure.

CONCLUSION

Percutaneous dilatational tracheostomy is safe and highly effective in well trained and experienced hands. Most of these contraindications should not be viewed as prohibitions, but as suggestions related to skill level and training of the operator. We have performed percutaneous tracheostomy in several relative contraindications by selecting a suitable PDT kit, monitoring, smaller incision, dissection of pretracheal tissue with or without bronchoscopic guidance. The patients may be chosen or rejected for the PDT on the basis of level of experience and safety record.

REFERENCES

1. Heffner JE, Miller KS, Sahn SA. Tracheostomy in the intensive care unit. Part 2: Complications. Chest 1986;90:430-6.
2. Mansharamani NG, Koziel H, Garland R, LoCicero 3rd J, Critchlow J, Ernst A. Safety of bedside percutaneous dilatational tracheostomy in obese patients in the ICU. Chest 2000;117:1426-9.
3. Meyer M, Critchlow J, Manasharamani N, Angel LF, Garland R, Ernst A. Repeat bedside percutaneous dilatational tracheostomy is a safe procedure. Crit Care Med 2002;30:986-8.
4. Friedman Y, Mayer AD. Bedside percutaneous tracheostomy in critically ill patients. Chest 1993; 104:532-5.
5. Freeman BD, Isabella K, Lin N, Buchman TG. A meta-analysis of prospective trials comparing percutaneous and surgical tracheostomy in critically ill patients. Chest 2000;118:1412-8.
6. Bass SP, Field LM. Repeat percutaneous tracheostomy. Anaesthesia 1994;49:649.
7. Mazzon D, Zanardo D, Dei Tos AP. Repeat percutaneous tracheostomy with the Ciaglia technique after translaryngeal tracheostomy. Intensive care Med 1999; 25:639.
8. Klein M, WEksler N, Kaplan DM, Weksler D, Chorny I, Gurman GM. Emergency percutaneous tracheostomy is feasible in experienced hands. Eur J Emerg Med 2004; 11:108-12.
9. Clarke J, Jaffery A. How we do it: Emergency percutaneous tracheostomy: A case series. Clin Otolaryngol Allied Sci 2004;29:558-61.
10. Ben-Nun A, Altman E, Best LA. Emergency percutaneous tracheostomy in trauma patients: An early experience. Ann Thorac Surg 2004;77:1045-7.
11. Ault MJ, Ault B, Ng PK. Percutaneous dilatational tracheostomy for emergent airway access. J Intensive care Med 2003;18:222-6.
12. Mazzon D, Zanatta P, Curtolo S, Bernardi V, Bosco E. Upper airway obstruction by retropharyngeal hematoma after cervical spine trauma. J Neurosurg Anesthesiol 1998;10:237-40.
13. Dob DP, McLure HA, Soni N. Failed intubation and emergency percutaneous tracheostomy. Anaesthesia 1998;53:72-4.
14. Toursarkissian B, Fowler CL, Zweng TN, Kearney PA. Percutaneous dilatational tracheostomy in children and teenagers. J Pediatr Surg 1994;29:1421-4.
15. Zawadzka-Glos L, Rawicz M, Chmielik M. Percutaneous tracheostomy in children. Int J Pediatr Otorhinolaryngol. 2004;68:1387-90.
16. Fantoni A, Ripamonti D. A non-derivative, non-surgical tracheostomy: The translaryngeal method. Intensive Care Med 1997;23:386-92.
17. Mayberry JC, Wu IC, Goldman RK, Chestnut RM. Cervical spine clearance and neck extension during percutaneous tracheostomy in trauma patients. Crit Care Med 2000;28:3436-40.
18. Sustc A, Krstulovic B, Eskinja N, Zelic M, Ledic D, Turina D. Surgical tracheostomy versus percutaneous dilational tracheostomy in patients with anterior cervical spine fixation: Preliminary report. Spine 2002;27: 1942-5.
19. Kluge S, Meyer A, Kuhnelt P, Baumann HJ, Kreymann G. Percutaneous tracheostomy is safe in patients with severe thrombocytopenia. Chest 2004;126:547-51.

Chapter 15

Percutaneous Tracheostomy versus Surgical Tracheostomy

Arturo Guarino, Guido Merli

INTRODUCTION

Tracheostomy is a procedure commonly performed on Intensive Care Unit (ICU) patients with the aim of avoiding a too long time of endotracheal translaryngeal intubation when airway control and mechanical ventilation are needed.

Open surgical tracheostomy (ST) was the only procedure known in past years and centuries. More recently, in 1985, thoracic surgeon P. Ciaglia[1] introduced Percutaneous Dilatational Tracheostomy (PDT), a new approach in which tracheostomy was performed by a multiple dilatators technique applying the well known Seldinger guide wire technique. It was considered an improvement of a previous percutaneous method proposed by Shelden in 1955, which used a cutting trocar, soon after abandoned because of the high incidence of complications.[2] During following years different techniques of percutaneous tracheostomy were proposed and introduced into clinical practice:[3-8] they now represent the first and most popular choice for performing tracheostomy in ICU. However, surgical tracheostomy remains the technique preferred by several authors and in many countries it represents the most chosen procedure of tracheotomy in ICU patients.[9-11]

A Difficult Comparison

A large medical literature has considered the question of comparing different tracheostomy techniques. So far there is not sufficient evidence to prove the superiority of one percutaneous technique compared to all the others. Moreover a great debate exists about the comparison among percutaneous and surgical techniques, especially considering perioperative and early and late postoperative complications. First of all we should consider that the comparison is not between two well standardized procedures but among different percutaneous and surgical techniques. Surgical tracheotomy is usually performed according to Jackson procedure described in 1909[12] but the scientific literature differs in operative details according to:

- Skin incision:
  - Vertical
  - Horizontal
- Dislodgment or ligature and resection of thyroid isthmus with consequent difference in site of tracheostomy:
  - Trans-isthmic between 2nd and 3rd tracheal ring
  - Sub-isthmic between 3rd and 4th tracheal ring

- Tracheal wall incision
  - Vertical
  - Horizontal
  - U-shaped flag technique
- Fixation to skin of the anterior tracheal wall with transfixed stitches

Seldinger technique is common to all percutaneous dilatational approaches, while the procedure used to perform tracheostomy can be different: either multistep dilational technique (PDT Ciaglia technique) or single dilator technique (Ciaglia Blue Rhino, Griggs GWDF, Frova Percu Twist, Ambesh T-Dagger) are used in clinical practice. The different structural and functional characteristics of the dilatators used in these techniques require different operative approaches and skin incision extents. Finally, Translaryngeal Tracheotomy (TLT) proposed by Fantoni is performed through retrograde approach with Seldinger maneuvre.

It is not clear what is the real influence of any of the above reported different techniques on the results and outcome of tracheostomy. Data from literature do not support specific procedural indications due to a lack of objective results. The lack of endoscope monitoring, reported by several studies, contributes to unclear results. Endoscopy must be considered a useful guidance to a well performed tracheal puncture in the midline, avoids paratracheal positioning of tracheostomy tubes, reduces the risks of posterior tracheal wall injuries, makes easier the learning curve of these techniques.[13-17] Further the use of Fiberoptic Bronchoscope (FOB) enables transillumination of neck soft tissues and often allows to recognize vessels running across neck midline: the change in puncture site or the preventive ligature of vessels may help in reducing the incidence of perioperative bleeding complications. We believe that another important role played by endoscopy is the discovering and the evaluation of possible injuries involving vocal cords, larynx and trachea. These damages can be present before tracheostomy, due

to translaryngeal intubation. Therefore, clinical studies comparing different tracheostomy techniques should consider the use of endoscope video assistance during percutaneous procedures.[18]

Most of the scientific papers of the last 20 years are observational studies and only few are prospective randomized controlled trials (RCT). This makes difficult, whenever impossible, an exact comparison of tracheotomy outcomes and a standardized classification of complications. In fact, some authors classify peri- and postoperative complications in mild, intermediate and severe; others report only complications considered clinically relevant. Severe complications are generally well defined and universally reported, while intermediate or mild complications are subjective, imprecisely described, not well detailed and their incidence is affected by the accuracy with which they are sought. For example, perioperative bleeding is evaluated following different parameters: millilitres of blood drained, number of gauzes, possibility of bleeding control by finger pressure, need of hemotransfusion or surgical hemostasis.

Peristomal infections are differently defined as well: cellulitis, local infection with purulent secretions, need of antibiotics, extension in millimetres of stoma infection, local necrosis, etc. Not homogeneous definitions cause confusing results. In a prospective and randomized study comparing ST and PDT, Holdgard et al[19] reported bleeding in 20% of PDT and 87% of ST patients, while stoma infection in 10% of PDT and 63% of ST patients. In another prospective and randomized study Porter and Ivatury[20] compared the two techniques and found 0% incidence of perioperative bleeding and stoma infection both in PDT and ST group.

Which is the best tracheostomy technique? Lack of evidence but a growing experience.

The potential benefits of PDT recognized by most of the sustainers of these techniques are listed in Table 15.1. Some of these advantages must be revaluated considering more recent literature data.

Percutaneous dilatational tracheostomy was firstly proposed as a procedure to be performed at the bedside of ICU patients: this characteristic avoids the risks related to the transport of critical patients from ICU to the operating theatre, reduces the costs related to the use of operatory rooms (OR), limits waiting times between decision making and the procedure, allowing a better and earlier timing of tracheostomy.[21] PDT successfully performed at the bedside of ICU patients suggested the opportunity to perform ST at the same place. Some studies demonstrated similar safety and efficacy of this maneuvre performed at the bedside compared to the or procedure.[9,10,20,22-24] Higher costs for ST are only related to operatory room expenses. It is obvious that if both procedures are equally performed in ICU, PDT is quite more expensive for the need of specific tools and FOB video assistance.

Table 15. 1: Advantages of PDT
• Bedside procedure • Easy performance • Rapid learning curve • Early timing of tracheostomy • Short operative time • Reduction of tissue trauma • Low cost

Some authors report a shorter operative time of PDT. We do not believe that operative time can be pointed as a factor of clinical relevance, especially if differences are limited to a 10-15 minutes time. However, data from literature (Table 15.2) show that both techniques have wide ranging operative times and, according to some studies, ST can even be faster than PDT.[10,28,30]

The authors generally agree about some contraindication to PDT (Table 15.3). Some of these contraindications are just absolute, like infection at local site, emergency, irregular neck anatomy, neck cancer or goitre, pulsing vessels above tracheostomy access, or factors causing difficulties in recognizing specific landmarks. Some other contraindications, once considered absolute, are now questioned. Over 20 years experience in PDT has potentially increased knowledge in clinical practice and operative approaches. In fact, according to some authors, PDT can be considered a safe procedure in obese patients, but others report a high incidence of severe complications.[15,32,33] The low number of patients enrolled in these surveys is not sufficient, however, to express a final assessment. In our limited experience with morbidly obese patients, a large amount of fatty tissue overlapping trachea made it impossible to reach

Table 15.2: PDT and ST operative time (min ± SD)			
Source		*PDT*	*ST*
Hazard[29]	(1991)	4.3 ± 2.2	13.5 ± 7.3
Friedman[25]	(1996)	8.2 ± 4.9	33.9 ± 14
Holdgaard[19]	(1998)	11.5 (7-24)	15.5 (5-47)
Gysin[30]	(1999)	18.2 ± 11.2	15.8 ± 5.5
Freeman[21]	(2001)	20.1 ± 2	41.7 ± 3.9
Antonelli[26]	(2005)	17 ± 10	22 ± 6
Melloni[27]	(2002)	14 ± 6	41.4 ± 14
Silvester[28]	(2006)	20 (15-30)	17 (15-20)
Levin[22]	(2001)	NA	27
Heikkinen[23]	(2000)	11 ± 6	14 ± 6
Massick[10]	(2001)	11 (4-18)	BS* 10(5-16); OR 16(10-27)
Goldenberg[31]	(2003)	5	20

* BS Bedside; OR Operatory room

Table 15.3: Contraindications to percutaneous dilatational tracheostomy

- Emergent tracheotomy
- Age < 12 years
- Inability to palpate cricoid
- Midline neck mass
- Enlarged thyroid
- Pulsating palpable blood vessel over the tracheotomy site
- Uncorrected coagulation disorder
- PEEP > 20 cm H_2O
- Increased intracranial pressure (relative)
- Obese short neck (relative)
- History of difficult intubations (relative)
- Fixation of cervical spine (relative)

the anterior tracheal wall with first-step dilator of the Ciaglia percutaneous kit in one case, and with the screw-type PercuTwist dilator in the second patient. We believe that PDT must be considered with great prudence in obese patients and ST should yet be viewed as the first choice and safer procedure.

Coagulative disorders initially contraindicated PDT, but this was later widely questioned. In a retrospective study Kluge et al reported low incidence of hemorrhagic complications after Griggs GWDF in 42 low platelet patients with PLT count < 52000/mm^2; only two patients were affected by major bleeding.[34] In case of hemorrhagic risk, other authors choose Fantoni TLT technique: they believe this procedure provides immediate tamponade at the site of tracheostomy.[35] However, most of prospective randomized studies usually exclude patients affected by coagulative disorders, therefore there is no evidence that one technique is superior in preventing bleeding in these patients. This matter is far from being solved and needs more studies and investigations.[10,21,26-28]

Only four meta-analysis comparing PDT and ST are present in scientific literature. Dulguerov et al.[36] examined both prospective and observational studies on a wide range of patients undergoing four different techniques of PDT; two of these techniques were later considered obsolete because

of the high rate of related complications. The authors found that tracheostomized patients were affected by a rate of perioperative complications, which resulted more frequent and severe, after PDT than after ST. Among postoperative complications, tracheal stenosis presents higher incidence after PDT than after recently performed surgical procedures. Finally, inside percutaneous dilatational techniques, the lower rate of complications was related to the use of progressive dilatation and to the presence of video-assistance with endoscope monitoring.

Two other meta-analysis were published in 2000 by Freeman et al and by Cheng et al.[37,38] These authors examined respectively five and four studies, among which four were cited by both meta analysis but only three were prospective randomized studies.[19,20,25,29,39] In all these studies PDT was performed according to Ciaglia's multi step dilatators technique. Both meta-analysis agree to consider PDT a faster procedure with lower incidence of perioperative bleeding. The incidence of postoperative complications, with particular respect to bleeding and wound infection, is lower after PDT. These authors believe that after PDT the tight adherence of tracheostoma which fits snugly around the tracheostomy tube and the mild trauma of soft tissues, with lack of dead space, are important factors to limit hemorrhage and to avoid infectious processes. None of the studies analyzed in these meta-analyses examined the late complications of PDT and ST.

In the last and more recent meta-analysis Delaney et al examined 17 randomized controlled trials highly selected.[40] These authors considered outcomes only when referred as clinically relevant, needing therapies or potentially life threatening. The conclusions of the meta-analysis partially agree with previous studies: PDT is related to a significant lower incidence of wound infections. Otherwise bleeding incidence seems to be lower after PDT, but there is no statistical significance. The other major early postoperative complications show no statistically significant differences between PDT and ST. Only a few of these studies examined late complications of tracheostomy, but the low number of patients admitted to the follow-up does not allow any definitive clinical assessment.

The incidence of late complications of tracheostomy, both PDT and ST, is matter of strong discussion because the data from literature are affected by extremely high variability and lack of agreement. Among the most clinically relevant late complications of tracheostomy they must be considered tracheal stenosis, tracheomalacia, late hemorrhage caused by tracheo innominate fistula, tracheoesophageal fistula (Table 15.4). Last two complications are extremely rare and show little or no correlation with the operative technique, PDT or ST: in fact their late onset is usually caused by the pressure of tracheal tube and/or its cuff on tracheal wall. Coexisting factors are the presence of the nasal-gastric tube, especially if maintained for a long time, some acute and severe illnesses like low responsive shock conditions, severe sepsis, local infections, immunodepression, and the prolonged dependence from mechanical ventilation.

More attention than in the past is now reserved to the esthetic result from tracheotomy scar. Recent studies confirm that better results are related to PDT, probably because of the reduced tissue trauma caused by this procedure, and mostly because of the lower incidence of postoperative stoma infections.[27,28,30]

The reported incidence of tracheal stenosis is quite variable, between 0% and 63% after PDT and between 0% and 96% after ST.[41-46] This high heterogeneity is clearly affected by different evaluations expressed in literature. Most studies considered stenosis of clinical relevance. Otherwise some follow-up reports analyzed both radiological imaging and bronchoscope views and discovered a high incidence of minor asymptomatic stenotic lesions, the so called radiological stenosis, involving just more than 10% of tracheal diameter. When stenoses are more extended and cause a reduction of tracheal diameter greater than 50% they become symptomatic only during exercise. In such cases reported incidence was lower. Finally, when stenoses are symptomatic at rest, they surely involve more than 75% of tracheal lumen[43,47,48].

A site related classification divides stenosis into high laryngeal (above, inside, below glottis), low laryngeal (cricoid), high tracheal (cervical trachea), low tracheal (intrathoracic trachea).[49] It's important to note that several factors play a relevant role in causing tracheal stenosis and tracheomalacia. Endotracheal translaryngeal intubation, which usually precede tracheostomy, may itself cause injury to laryngotracheal structures: involving mechanisms are the direct trauma during manoeuvres, the pressure caused by endotracheal tube and by its cuff upon different portions of laryngeal and tracheal mucosa, the size and materials of endotracheal tubes, the tractions of ventilatory lines, the time of intubation, the presence of infective complications. Following mechanisms are the direct and indirect injuries caused by tracheostomy; any loss of integrity in tracheal wall, just weakened by a long time intubation, can further damage cartilaginous structures and potentially cause bacterial super-infections.

Table 15.4: Long-term complications of tracheostomy		
Minor	*Intermediate*	*Major*
Granuloma	Late hemorrhage	Tracheal stenosis
Unesthetic scar	Tracheostomy tube	Tracheomalacia
Persistent stoma	occlusion	Tracheoinnominate fistula
Severe hoarseness	Swallowing impairments	Tracheoesophageal fistula

In ST wide tissue opening and dissection are direct causes of the high incidence of infections; in fact tissue dissection modifies local microcirculation of cartilaginous rings, with following ischemia, necrosis and finally loss of tissues thickness.

PDT can prevent some of these complications; it is limited to a transcutaneous puncture and to a few millimetres skin incision without tissue dissection, it does not remove portions of tracheal rings and usually respects the integrity of the cartilaginous structure. The risks of infective processes are so really reduced. However, some anatomopathological studies demonstrated that PDT can also be a cause of injury to tracheal wall.[50-52] Cartilaginous rings fracture during PDT is a complication frequently reported in literature; its incidence, indicated by endoscope monitoring during PDT procedure, is widely lower than that 87% discovered by anatomopathologic studies.[52]

We must finally remember that there is paucity of data that correlate cartilaginous rings fracture to the risk of stenotic complications. A recent study, performed on a population of patients who underwent tracheal resection surgery for symptomatic tracheal stenosis, points out a relevant difference among injuries following PDT and ST.[53] The authors found that most of stenoses (58%) were sited in the subglottic space after PDT and at a 3-4 cm distance from vocal folds after ST. Different site of stenotic complications is probably direct consequence of a too high tracheal puncture during PDT performance. These authors finally consider the severity of this complication directly related to the high difficulty of performing surgery at cricoid level.

CONCLUSIONS

After first Ciaglia experience, in 1985, PDT gained an improving popularity during the following years. The development of new devices and the introductions of new techniques contributed to the creation of a 20 years experience in PDT, which is now the most commonly performed tracheostomy technique in ICU patients.

Intensivists and anesthetists mostly perform PDT in ICU. Otorhinolaryngologists, thoracic surgeons and other surgeons firstly looked at PDT with scepticism, but during last years they began to appreciate the advantages of PDT and to use it as an alternative to classic open ST. However, many operators prefer ST, which must be considered the technique of first choice in emergency conditions, in pediatric patients, in morbidly obesity, in case of neck or thyroid tumors, or in coagulative disorders. Not all these contraindications to PDT are surely absolute, but in some critically ill patients PDT is at high risk and conversion from PDT into ST is not infrequent. In case of little or no experience in surgical technique the rapid availability of one surgical team should be carefully planned.

Though PDT is known as an easy and fast technique, experience is however absolutely necessary, as for many other medical procedures. Video endoscope assistance reduces the incidence of perioperative complications, some of which can be severe. Video endoscopic monitoring must be considered not a useful complement but a necessary component throughout the whole procedure of percutaneous tracheostomy. Bedside PDT was firstly considered not only a clinical choice but also an economic and organizative advantage. Several experiences in recent years, however, showed that both PDT and ST can be performed in ICU with similar efficacy, safety and risks. It is just recognized that PDT has the advantage of ensuring a reduction in postoperative bleeding and in stoma infection with a best esthetic result of scar in respect with ST.

There are no data suggesting which procedure has the lower incidence of severe perioperative complications. Lastly follow-up data concerning late complications are poorly significant because of the lack of current homogenous recordings. PDT and ST will live together for many years again: they will both be performed with the aim of offering to patients the best operative procedure according to their clinical conditions, operator's capability and experience, with the lower rate of risks. This will be the future until one of them, PDT or ST, will be surely recognized better than the other one.

REFERENCES

1. Ciaglia P, Firsching R. Syniec C. Elective percutaneous dilatational tracheostomy. A new simple bedside procedure; preliminary report. Chest 1985;87:715-9.
2. Shelden C, Pudenz RH, Freshwater DB, Crue BL. A new method for tracheotomy. J Neurosurg 1995;12:428-31).
3. Schachner A, Ovil Y, Sidi J, Rogev M, Heilbronn Y, Levy M. Percutaneous tracheostomy: A new method. Crit Care Med 1989;17:1052-6.
4. Griggs WM, Werthley LIG, Gilligan JE, Thomas PD, Myburgh JA. A simple percutaneous tracheostomy technique. Surg Gynecol Obstet 1990;170:543-5.
5. Fantoni A, Ripamonti D. A non-derivative, non surgical tracheostomy: The translaryngeal method. Intensive Care Med 1997;23:386-92.
6. Ciaglia P. Technique, Complications and improvements in percutaneous dilatational tracheostomy. Chest 1999;115:1229-30.
7. Frova G, Quintel M. A new simple method for percutaneous tracheostomy: Controlled rotating dilation. A preliminary report. Intensive Care Med 2002; 28:299-303.
8. Ambesh SP, Tripathi M, Pandey CK, Pant KC, Singh PH. Clinical evaluation of the "T-Dagger™: A new bedside percutaneous dilational tracheostomy device. Anaesthesia 2005;60:708-11.
9. Wang SJ, Sercaz JA, Blackwell KE, Aghamohammadi MB, Wang MB. Open bedside tracheotomy in the intensive care unit. Laryngoscope 1999;109:891-3.
10. Massick DD, Yao S, Powell DM, Griesen D, Hobgood T, Allen JN, Schuller DE. Bedside tracheostomy in the intensive care unit: A prospective randomized trial comparing open surgical tracheostomy with endoscopically guided percutaneous dilational tracheotomy. Laryngoscope 2001;111:494-500.
11. Blot F, Melot C. Indications, timing and techniques of tracheostomy in 152 French ICUs. Chest 2005; 127:1347-52.
12. Jackson C. Tracheotomy. Laryngoscope 1909;18:285-90.
13. Marelli D, Paul A, Manolidis S, Walsh D, Odim JN, Burdon TA, Shennib H, Vestweber KH, Fleiszer DM, Mulder DS. Endoscopic guided percutaneous tracheostomy: Early results of a consecutive trial. J Trauma 1990;30:433-5.
14. Winkler WB, Karnik R, Seelmann O, Havlicek J, Slany J. Bedside percutaneous tracheostomy with endoscopic guidance: Experience with 71 ICU patients. Intensive Care Med 1994;20:476-9.
15. Barba CA, Angood PB, Kauder DR, Latenser B, Martin K, McGonigal MD, Phillips GR, Rotondo MF, Schwab CW. Broncoscopic guidance makes percutaneous tracheostomy a safe, cost-effective, and easy-to-teach procedure. Surgery 1995;118:879-83.
16. Ciaglia P. Video-assisted endoscopy, not just endoscopy for percutaneous dilatational tracheostomy. Chest 1999;115:915-6.
17. Polderman KH, Spijkstra JJ, deBree R, Christiaans HMT, Gelissen HPM, Wester JPJ, Girbes ARJ. Percutaneous dilatational tracheostomy in the ICU–Optimal organization, low complication rates, and description of a new complication. Chest 2003;123:1595-602.
18. Kost KM. Endoscopic percutaneous dilatational tracheotomy: A prospective evaluation of 500 consecutive cases. Laryngoscope 2005;115:1-30.
19. Holdgaard HO, Pedersen J, Jensen RH, Outzen KE, Midtgaard T, Johansen LV, Moller J. Paaske PB. Percutaneous dilatational tracheostomy versus conventional surgical tracheostomy. A clinical randomised study. Acta Anaesthesiol Scand 1998;42:545-50.
20. Porter JM, Ivatury RR. Preferred route of tracheostomy-percutaneous versus open at the bedside: A randomised, prospective study in the surgical intensive care unit. Am Surg 1999;65:142-6.
21. Freeman BD, Isabella K, Cobb JP, Boyle WA, Schmieg RE, Koleff MH, Lin N, Saak T, Thompson EC, Buchman TG. A prospective, randomised study comparing percutaneous with surgical tracheostomy in critically ill patients. Crit Care Med 2001;29:926-30.
22. Levin R, Trivikram L. Cost/benefit analysis of open tracheotomy, in the OR and at the bedside, with percutaneous tracheotomy. Laryngoscope 2001;111:1169-73.
23. Heikkinen M, Aarnio P, Hannukainen J. Percutaneous dilational tracheostomy or conventional surgical tracheostomy? Crit Care Med 2000;28:1399-402.
24. Bernard AC, Kenady DE. Conventional surgical tracheostomy as the preferred method of airway management. J Oral Maxillofac Surg 1999;57:310-5.
25. Friedman Y, Fildes J, Mizock B, Samuel J, Patel S, Appavu S, Roberts R. Comparison of percutaneous and surgical tracheostomy. Chest 1996;110:480-5.

26. Antonelli M, Michetti V, Di Palma A, Conti G, Pennisi MA, Arcangeli A, Montini L, Bocci MG, Bello G, Almadori G, Paludetti G, Proietti R. Percutaneous translaryngeal versus surgical tracheostomy: A randomized trial with 1-yr double-blind follow-up. Crit Care Med 2005;33:1015-20.

27. Melloni G, Muttini S, Gallioli G, Carretta A, Cozzi S, Gemma M, Zannini P. Surgical tracheostomy versus percutaneous dilatatinal tracheostomy. A prospective-randomized study with long-term follow-up. J Cardiovasc Surg (Torino)2002;43:113-21.

28. Silvester W, Goldsmith D, Uchino S, Bellomo R, Knight S, Seevanayagam S, Brazzale D, McMahon M, Buckmaster J, Hart GK, Opdam H, Pierce RJ, Gutteridge GA. Percutaneous versus surgical tracheostomy: A randomized controlled study with long-term follow-up. Crit Care Med 2006;34:2145-52.

29. Hazard P, Jones C, Benitone J. Comparative clinical trial of standard operative tracheostomy with percutaneous tracheostomy. Crit Care Med 1991;19:1018-24.

30. Gysin C, Dulguerov P, Guyot JP, Perneger TV, Abajo B, Chevrolet JC. Percutaneous versus surgical tracheostomy – A double-blind randomized trial. Ann Surg 1999;230:708-14.

31. Goldenberg D, Golz A, Huri A, Netzer A, Joachims HZ, Bar-Lavie Y. Percutaneous dilation tracheotomy versus surgical tracheotomy: Our experience. Otolaryngol Head Neck Surg 2003;128:358-63.

32. Mansharamani NG, Koziel H, Garland R LoCicero J, Ernst A. Safety of bedside percutaneous tracheostomy in obese patients in the ICU. Chest 2000;117: 1426-9.

33. Byhahn C, Lischke V, Meininger D, Halbig S, Westphal K. Peri-operative complications during percutaneous tracheostomy in obese patients. Anaesthesia 2005;60:12-5.

34. Kluge S, Meyer A, Kuhnelt P, Baumann HJ, Kreymann G. Percutaneous tracheostomy is safe in patients with severe thrombocypenia. Chest 2004;126:547-51.

35. Bardell T, Drover JW. Recent developments in percutaneous tracheostomy: Improving techniques and expanding roles. Curr Opin Crit Care. 2005;11:326-32

36. Dulguerov P, Gysin C, Perneger TV, Chevrolet J-C. Percutaneous or surgical tracheostomy: A meta-analysis. Crit Care Med 1999;27:1617-25.

37. Freeman BD, Isabella K, Lin N, Buchman TG. A Meta-analysis of prospective trials comparing percutaneous and surgical tracheostomy in critically ill patients. Chest 2000;118:1412-8.

38. Cheng E, Fee WE. Dilatational versus standard tracheostomy: A metaanalysis. Ann Otol Rhinol Laryngol 2000;109:803-7.

39. Crofts SL, Alzeer A, McGuire GP, Wong DT, Charles D. A comparison of precutaneous and operative tracheostomies in intensive care patients. Can J Anaesth 1995;42:775-9.

40. Delaney A, Bagshaw S, Nalos M. Percutaneous dilatational tracheostomy versus surgical tracheostomy in critically ill patients: A systematic review and a metaanalysis. Critical Care 2006;10:R55.

41. Winkler WB, Karnick R, Seelmann O, Havlicek J, Slany J. Bedside percutaneous dilational tracheostomy with endoscopic guidance: Experience with 71 ICU patients. Int Care Med 1994;20:476-9.

42. Marelli D, Paul A, Manolidis S, Walsh G, Odim JNK, Burdon TA, Shennib H, Vestweber KH, Fleiszer DM, Mulder DSl. Endoscopic guided percutaneous tracheostomy: Early results of a consecutive trial. J Trauma 1990;30:433-5.

43. Dollner R, Verch M, Schweiger P, Deluigi C, Graf P, Wallner F. Laryngotracheoscopic findings in long-term follow-up after Griggs tracheostomy. Chest 2002;122:206-12.

44. Skaggs JA,Cogbill CL. Tracheostomy: Management, mortality, complications. Am Surg 1969;35:393-6.

45. Dayal VS, El Masri W. Tracheostomy in the intensive care setting. Laryngoscope 1986;96:58-60.

46. Davidson IA,Cruickshank AN, Duthie WH et al. Lesions of the trachea following tracheostomy and endotracheal intubation. Proc R Soc Med 1971;64:886-92.

47. Van Heurn LWE, Goei R, de Ploeg I, Ramsay G, Brink PRG. Late complications of percutaneous dilatational tracheotomy. Chest 1996;110:1572-6.

48. Norwood S, Vallina Van L, Short K, Saigusa M, Fernandez LG, McLarty JW. Incidence of tracheal stenosis and other late complications after percutaneous tracheostomy. Ann Surg 2000;232:233-41.

49. Frova G, Guarino A. Le complicanze a distanza della tracheo(s)tomia. Anest Rianim Intens 1994;15: 322-6.

50. Hotchkiss KS, McCaffrey JC. Laryngotracheal injury after percutaneous dilational tracheostomy in cadaver specimens. Laryngoscope 2003;113:16-20.

51. Stoeckli SJ, Breitbach T, Schmid S. A clinical and histologic comparison of percutaneous dilational versus conventional surgical tracheostomy. Laryngoscope 1997;107:1643-6.

52. Van Heurn LWE, Theunissen P, Ramsay G, Brink P. Pathologic changes of the trachea after percutaneous dilatational tracheotomy. Chest 1996;109:1466-9.

53. Raghuraman G, Rajan S, Marzouk JK, Mullhi D, Smith F. Is tracheal stenosis caused by percutaneous tracheostomy different from that by surgical tracheostomy? Chest 2005;127:879-85.

Chapter 16

How to Judge a Tracheostomy: A Reliable Method of Comparison of the Different Techniques

Antonio Fantoni

If one made an unbiased examination of the studies published up to now on the various techniques of tracheostomy, one might not help noticing that the criteria used to evaluate a tracheostomy are greatly inappropriate, as there has been no uniformity in measured parameters and risk factors.

Studies evaluating the tracheostomy techniques have generally reported the number of patients, the pathology that required this procedure, the length of previous tracheal intubation and the list of complications. No data are given of the technical difficulties met in each patient and counted in a global score related to the entire series, so that usual judgment, grounded on the frequency and severity of the complications, is of no meaning. Even more astounding is the situation when a comparison is made, since, in this case, a superiority is given to the method that simply reports a lower number of complications. To create a certain reliability of the studies it is evidently indispensable to introduce the necessary remedies and adjust the way of looking at the problem.

Clearly Describe the Technique Used and Its Variations

Of the two basic techniques to accomplish a tracheostomy, surgical and percutaneous, the first is practized following a scheme remained unchanged over a century, while the latter can be carried out with numerous different techniques. In addition, one has to consider that each percutaneous technique has, in their turn, a few variations, elaborated by some users with the aim of adding improvements to the original version.

For instance, the PDT acronym indicates many versions of the original Ciaglia method which differ for various kinds of needle and wire insertion, for various shapes of the dilators and for the use or non use of bronchoscopy. The same situation can be observed with TLT as well. Some variations have not even been signalled in literature, which we came to acknowledge through personal communication or by chance. Since each of these variations may bear their own pros and cons, it is evident that, in comparative studies, these variations should be clearly illustrated in detail so that the reader can properly interpret the result and understand the cause of the complications which might occur.

The appearance of TLT, a new, contra-current technique, created the necessity to distinguish the percutaneous method into two categories according to the modality of the dilation: on the one hand, TLT with the inside/outside dilation, on the other, all the others with the outside/inside way. We deemed suitable to gather all the techniques of the second group under the same acronym OIT (Outside/Inside Tracheostomy), so as to make the exposition clearer and to underline their common drawback, the forced insertion of the tools into the trachea.

Get Accustomed to Looking into the Single Fractions of the Procedure

Having observed that every type of tracheostomy can be sectioned into three clear-cut phases (Table 16.1)[1], we have adopted this subdivision that allows one to analyze in detail, step by step, every single technique of tracheostomy.

The main advantage of this subdivision is the possibility to trace the pathogenesis of the occurred complications, giving them a precise time frame. Knowing that hemorrhages or tracheal lesions are originated in Phases 1, 2 or 3 is much more informative than what can be said by a mere list of complications.

Another significant advantage is represented by the possibility of carrying out more thorough comparisons, by opposing two different techniques phase by phase. It may be interesting to know the duration, the difficulty, and the risk of each phase. The importance of comparing the effects of the dilation procedure in TLT and in any other OITs on the anterior and posterior tracheal wall, is extremely clear in (Fig. 16.1).

In the (Fig. 16.2), is shown the very different result in making a hole in soft plastic material by using the specific punch or a simple awl. There is a deep analogy with what happen in TLT and in OITs: only the two opposite pressures, exclusively achievable with the inside/outside dilation, can ensure a precise, non-frayed stoma.

Furthermore, the adoption of the subdivision helps to introduce new concepts in the comparative studies. In every technique one can spot a phase that characterizes the method, generally represented in phase 2 by the modality of the dilation maneuvres. On the other hand, there are phases of different

Table 16.1 The subdivision into phases of tracheostomies			
Phase	*1*	*2*	*3*
Surgical Tracheostomy (ST)	tissue dissection	trachea opening	cannula insertion
Outside/Inside Tracheostomy (OIT)	needle insertion	dilation	cannula insertion
Translaryngeal Tracheostomy (TLT)	needle insertion	dilation	cannula inversion

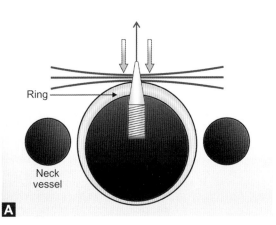

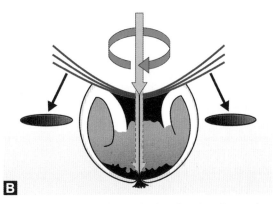

Ring

Neck vessel

A　　　　　　**B**

Fig. 16.1: Different effects of TLT (left) and OITs (right) on the anterior and posterior tracheal wall and neck vessels

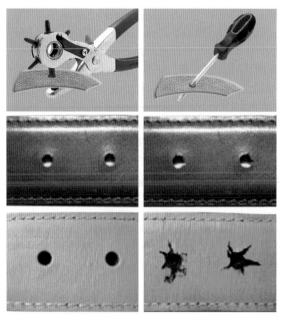

Fig. 16.2: Different results with different technique of making a hole in plastic material or leather

techniques quite overlapping. For instance, all the OITs recognize the same modality of needle and guide wire insertion and thus, in a hypothetical comparison between Blue Rhino and Griggs method (to cite a case), the complications of Phase 1 should not be considered since they depend exclusively on the expertise of the operator, not on the technique per se.

Regarding the variations of TLT, they have an identical Phase 2, but the substantial differences of Phases 1 and 3 have considerable consequences on the level of safety and, therefore, on the extension of the range of contraindications of each variation.

Register all the Useful Clinical Information about the Patient

Report the Essential Anatomical Data of the Neck

A trained eye can recognize "difficult tracheostomy" from afar. Yet, the warning given by observing a short and stout neck can be translated into the clinical documentation by registering the neck circumference and the crico-sternal notch distance, related to the height and weight of the patient. The checking of the specific landmarks of the neck is another essential point for the whole valuation, being well know that all OITs are considered contraindicated when these important clinical signs are obscured. Obviously, the data should be derived from each patient, indexed and collected to create a global score of the whole series of cases, the only means of performing sound comparisons.

Consider the Respiratory Function

One of the most important prerequisites of a technique of tracheostomy is the ability to grant an adequate respiratory support. Not all the methods are able to ensure this performance and thus, many of them are quite contraindicated to the patient with the heavier impairment of the lung. An ARDS patient needs high PIP and PEEP which can be supplied only if there is a circuit with perfect sealing in all of its parts, starting from the connection between the various kinds of tubes and natural airway. Accidental or a scheduled interruption of the ventilation and the continuous distending pressure, gives way to a rapid pulmonary collapse, shunts and intense desaturation.

For general consensus all the OITs are contraindicated to patients requiring PEEP > 10 cm H_2O and not having stable and effective respiratory system. In the basic TLT, the use of the rigid cuffed tracheoscope in Phase 1 and of the cuffed ventilation catheter in Phases 2 and 3, ensures the continuity of an adequate tidal volume and PEEP along the entire procedure to whichever type of patient. On the contrary, some TLT variations are not equally fitting to comply with the respiratory requirements of the most challenging cases.

Indeed, it does seem unbelievable that this important component of the global difficulty occurring during a tracheostomy is generally quite neglected.

Note the Difficulty of the Airway Access

It is enough to think of the problems created by cranio-facial abnormalities to the endoscopy and respiratory control, sometimes so exasperated as to discourage the carrying out of a percutaneous procedure, to understand how the omission of this data may weight on the comparison.

Register the Tracheal Condition before the Tracheostomy

The consequences of the preliminary tracheal intubation may be very different, and are related only partially to the duration of the intubation. We observed cases of massive damage of the trachea after a few hours of intubation and a normal aspect of the mucosa after twenty days. On these results, the adoption of a very soft tube, as small as possible, and the quality of nursing exert a prevailing influence. No humidification of the gases, continuous tractions on the tube, hyperinflation of the cuff are the main causes of an unsuccessful outcome. Heavy inflammation of the tracheal wall, fibrin layers reducing the lumen and creating obstructive flaps bring to a substantial increase of the risk of complications in all the steps of the tracheostomy, from needle to cannula insertion. Therefore, we conclude that the prior detailed picture of the conditions of the trachea is much more meaningful than knowing how many days the intubation lasted.

Adopt the Standard Evaluation of the Occurred Complications

The evaluation of a tracheostomy technique and the comparisons suffer from the relative paucity of the most severe complication, like tracheoeso-phageal fistula, major bleeding, cardiac arrest and death that makes it rather difficult to establish true superiority. Furthermore, looking over the specific literature, it is easy to agree on the total absence of homogeneity in the choice and evaluation of the complications of the tracheostomies. Some of them are not complications, but only difficulties, some others are events not related to the technique of tracheostomy. Frequently, the complications are underestimated. To give an example, considering a bruising of the posterior tracheal wall like a small drawback, is not correct, if we consider that between bruising and laceration or perforation there is only pure luck. Indeed, the weight of these complications is much more consistent as it demonstrates that technique has brought the operator closer to a major incident.

In this situation a noteworthy step forward, would be to follow an opposite approach, by taking into greater account all the clinical signs generally considered of no importance, like a small blood loss, short desaturations, small mucosal tears of the trachea, ring fractures, therefore considering them precious sentinels of what might have been more severe.

The Pitfall of the Pre-selection of the Patients

With the exclusion of the more challenging cases the overall incidence of complications is remarkably lowered, making the comparison much less sensible. Pre-selection hampers ST and TLT which don't have all the contraindications of OITs.

Just from the beginning, the comparisons between surgical and Ciaglia tracheostomies were always performed with exclusion of the most challenging patients, contraindicated only to PDT. And, on the base of a mere global count of the complications, it was concluded that "PDT appeared to be superior to the conventional tracheostomy", despite.

- The excluded patients underwent ST
- If difficulties raised during PDT, conversion to ST was performed
- The more severe intraprocedural complications occurred with PDT.

As regard the widespread opinion of the superiority of the PDT over the surgical tracheostomy (ST) some authors declared that ST, if performed by a skilful operator, has fewer risks and is practically without contraindications.[2] Also in my personal experience on three hundred STs in adults and 46 in pediatric patients, this opinion is confirmed: I never had to rush into an operating theatre for an emergency.

Examine the Surgical Component of a Technique

Starting from the premise that the great majority of the intensivists don't have a particular proficiency in surgery, it appear obvious that a percutaneous technique with a smaller component of invasive maneuvres (skin incision, blunt dissection with forceps of the pretracheal layers, vessel ligature), should have a higher score in the comparative studies.

Do Not Consider Unrelated Complications

It is wrong to include in the list of complications some postprocedural events not directly dependent on the type of tracheostomy technique, such as accidental decannulation, which is strictly dependent on the nursing, not on the type of tracheostomy. With a high level of assistance, the frequency of the decannulation is very low. In our unit, since over 30 years, all the patients on controlled ventilation are submitted to supine-prone positioning, that we consider mandatory in every form of respiratory failure, including the cases of neurological patients with normal lungs at the beginning of the treatment. In a thousand patients, thanks to the great dedication of the staff to this procedure, the problem of accidental decannulation has not been felt with any kind of tracheostomy.

A second example of these incongruities is the attribution of a tracheal decubitus caused by the cannula to a particular tracheostomy technique. This complication that may bring about a complete

tearing of the posterior tracheal wall is commonly due to a rigid device, kept tipped caudally for a long time and may occur with every type of method.

Don't make confusion between the terms difficult and new procedure.

TLT is a quite novel method that contradicts the traditional concepts to make a tracheostomy. Therefore, it is obvious that some steps are unusual and demand a special training. However, they are neither complex nor difficult.[3,4] Indeed, after a short training, one realizes it is simpler and safer to extract a cannula in TLT than to insert dilator and cannula in OITs.

Consider the Rate of Ring Fracture as a Reliable Index of Local Trauma

A precise, sensible measure of the local tissue trauma caused by a tracheostomy technique is represented by the rate of ring fractures it produces. These complications must not be under evaluated since they are always the cause of internal bleeding, mucosal flap, and obstructive crises with cartilaginous stumps dislocation.

Among the various methods, the greatest percentage is showed by the single-step dilation techniques, due to the rough pushing or rotating force of the instruments. A remarkable contributory factor of ring damage is represented by the insertion of the cannula, for the harmful dragging of the neck anatomical layers into the tracheal lumen. In TLT, the two opposite pressure, by fingers and cone, protect the ring and permit to achieve a pure ring divarication that, together with the lack of the insertion maneuvre of the cannula, offers a virtual absence of ring fractures.

Count the Percentage of Contraindications among the Most Important Criteria to Evaluate the Intrinsic Safety of a Technique

A technique can be defined intrinsically safe if it doesn't involve dangerous maneuvres, for skilful operators as well. The proscription of a technique in a certain kind of patient takes origin from the recurrences of determined unwanted events with that particular technique in those particular patients.

Pushing pointed tools into the trachea is the most typical example, the weak point of all OITs that keeps provoking tracheal lesions also in qualified centres, despite the mandatory application of the endoscopic control. The lack of a closed respiratory system does not ensure ventilation with high PIP and PEEP during the tracheostomy, so that ARDS patients should be excluded.

In OITs, tearing and jagging of the peristomal tissue and the fractures of the tracheal rings, caused by the indrawing or rotating dragging forces of instruments, expose to bleeding complications and therefore, rule out all the patients with severe coagulopathies. TLT for the minimal trauma and its efficient respiratory support is considered the most suitable technique for these kind of very challenging cases.[5,6]

Another source of contraindication is the rough insertion of dilators and cannula from outside into a small and very collapsible trachea of a child as in OITs, while, on the contrary, the inside/outside direction of the dilation and the absence of a true insertion of a cannula, make TLT the right method for pediatric cases.

CONCLUSIONS

Tracheostomy is a valuable component in the area of respiratory assistance, but it becomes a substantial cause of the patient's unfavorable outcome if it entails too many severe complications. The need of reliable comparisons, so as to permit sounder choices, is evident. Our present study contains some suggestions that allow us to accomplish evaluations much more thorough and exacting than that one used, or not used at all, up to now.

Simplistic, misleading comparisons must not be accepted any longer. If you start filling in a data base form, you will notice the advantage of having precious information available to implement a precise score of difficulties for each patient and for the whole competing series.

The adoption of these new criteria would avoid unbelievable mistakes like the magnification over fourteen years of Ciaglia method, defined simple, safe, and cost effective, the technique of choice for routine elective tracheostomy.[7] In spite of this, in 1999, the author himself [8], under the weight of a numberless reports of tracheal lesions, declared "The day of the rigid dilators in PDT is over" because the risk of tracheal damage from the use of rigid dilators is unacceptable.

REFERENCES

1. Fantoni A. Nuovi criteri di comparazione: le fasi della tracheostomia e i dati anatomici essenziali. Minerva Anestesiol 2004;70:445-8.
2. Porter JM, Ivatury RR. Preferred route of tracheostomy-Percutaneous versus open at the bedside: A randomized, prospective study in the surgical intensive care unit. Am Surgeon 1999;65:142-6.
3. Konopke R, Zimmerman T, Volk - A, et al. Prospective evaluation of retrograde percutaneous translaryngeal tracheostomy (Fantoni procedure): Technique and results of the Fantoni tracheostomy in a surgical intensive care unit. Head & Nek 2006;28:355-9.
4. Adam H, Hemprich A, Kock C, et al. Safety and practicability of percutaneous translaryngeal tracheotomy (Fantoni technique) in surgery of maxillofacial and oropharyngeal tumors. Own results and review of literature. J Cranio –Maxillofacial Surgery 2008;36:3846.
5. Byhahn C, Lischke V, Westphal K. Translaryngeal tracheostomy in highly unstable patients. Anaesthesia 2000;55:678-82.
6. Milligan KR, McCollum JC. Translaryngeal tracheostomy in high-risk patient. Anaesthesia 2000; 55:1132.
7. Ciaglia P and KD Graniero. Percutaneous dilatational tracheostomy. Results and long-term follow-up. Chest 1992;101:464-7.
8. Ciaglia P: Technique, complications, and improvements in percutaneous dilatational tracheostomy. Chest 1999; 115:1229-30.

Chapter 17

The Need to Compare Different Techniques of Tracheostomy in More Reliable Way

Antonio Fantoni

In 1985 Ciaglia introduced his method of percutaneous tracheostomy (PDT) based on the use of multiple dilators[1] that has rapidly gained widespread acceptance in everyday clinical practice and in literature. An endless number of papers followed, illustrating the new technique as a huge breakthrough and its superiority over surgical tracheostomy (ST).

In 1999, just after 14 years, Ciaglia announced that the rigid dilators were too dangerous and thus, they must be banned. He wrote: "The day of the rigid dilators is over".[2] It is rather strange that this statement, an actual rejection of his method, was said after such a long period of continuous hailing of its benefits. The most convincing interpretation of this about-turn cannot be very far from the large number of mentions of the injuries of the posterior tracheal wall, reported in literature, and, even more so, of a greater number of unpublished cases, that came to light by chance or by personal communication.[3]

We imported the PDT in our country in 1991 through the first Italian study,[4] but very soon we discovered that the danger of tracheal lesion was always possible even with skilful operators, and therefore the method was abandoned well ahead of time, exactly seven years before the announcement by Ciaglia. Therefore, we wonder why, at least, why the emphasis on the safety of this technique was not shortened a long time earlier?

This situation can only be explained by the fact that the criteria currently used are not reliable, and authorize whoever to affirm that his method is the best of all. If we are going to examine these criteria, we can easily find out the following incongruities:

First: The studies on the tracheostomy are usually lacking in data about the anatomical features of the neck, essential for giving a precise evaluation of the difficulties that the operator is going to face. Apart from some anecdotal mentions about a "short and stout neck", generally made by the attempt to justify an intraprocedural complication, detailed information of the neck, at least the circumference and the crico-sternal distance related to height and weight of the patient, are not registered at all.

Second: No mention is made of the difficulties of the laryngeal approach that may create serious problems during the various steps of the procedure, from the preparatory intubation to endoscopic and respiratory control.

Third: The descriptions of the conditions of the trachea before tracheostomy are never reported. Inflammatory reaction, edema, fibrin deposition narrow the lumen and weaken the tracheal wall, making the insertion of the needle more difficult and the dilation and the introduction of the cannula more dangerous. Having observed many cases of severe damage of the trachea after a few hours of translaryngeal intubation, we estimate that the detailed picture of the conditions of the trachea before the tracheostomy is much more meaningful than knowing how many days the intubation lasted.

Fourth: There is a big difference between normal and ARDS patients in performing a tracheostomy. In severe acute respiratory failure, the need of maintaining adequate ventilation with high PIP and PEEP, requires a perfect sealing of the respiratory system, not achievable with every kind of procedure. In these patients, also a short period of obstruction, caused by the presence of the fiberscope in the endotracheal tube, or of big dilators in the tracheal lumen and the aleatory sealing of the circuit, could result in being rather harmful. Despite the fact that the respiratory conditions can remarkably influence the difficulties of tracheostomy, this issue was completely ignored in up-to-day comparisons.

Fifth: Another incongruity is represented by the common habit of comparing groups of patients after having excluded the most challenging cases, like patients with a particularly stocky neck, with an impossible location of external markers, with uncorrectable coagulopathies, which require undue force by the insertion of tools or the need of high PIP and PEEP, pediatric patients, namely all the cases contraindicated for percutaneous methods with a general consensus.

The preselection reduces the value of the comparison for the two basic mechanisms. When the techniques under examination have the same contraindications, the selection does not obviously alter the comparison, but it is equally misleading for both methods since it reduces the rate of complications, especially of the more severe ones that have the greatest influence on the acceptance or the rejection of a tracheostomy technique. On the contrary, when there are remarkable differences of the range of indications, the pre-selection is like a car competition with evident differences of performance and imposing a low speed limit. The

finish line is crossed at the same time by the contenders, making it impossible for an absolute winner to come up. This is the situation when a percutaneous technique is compared to surgical tracheostomy. Several studies completed in the past concluded that the percutaneous method appeared to be superior to conventional tracheostomy[5,6] even if, ironically, the excluded patients underwent ST and converting percutaneous into ST was regularly practised if difficulties were raised during the procedure in the selected cases.

Working only on easy patients, less safe methods are clearly privileged because, the group of patients which would have enormously increased the number and severity of their complications, is withdrawn. According to some authors,[7] if ST is performed by skilful operators it has fewer risks and is practically without contraindications. Also with our past experience on three hundred STs in adults and 46 in pediatric patients, this is confirmed: we never had to rush into an operating theatre for an emergency. Moreover, we observed that also the incidence of stomite, considered a typical and frequent complication of ST, that has unfavourably influenced the result of the previous comparisons ST/percutaneous, can be markedly reduced by a good surgeon with a small opening in the neck.

And then, the large diffusion of percutaneous methods should be attributed not so much to greater safety but to less invasivity than ST, which allows even an intensivist with a scarce surgical expertise to perform a tracheostomy, without been accused of turf encroachment.

The appearance of TLT, a new, contra-current technique,[8,9] created the necessity to distinguish the percutaneous method into two groups according to the modality of the dilation: on the one hand, TLT with the inside/outside dilation, on the other, all the others with the outside/inside way. We deemed suitable to gather all the techniques of the second group under the same acronym OIP (outside/inside percutaneous), so as to make the exposition clearer and especially, because they have substantially the same drawbacks from the common handicap, the forced insertion of the tools into the trachea. A recent article just emphasised that the major advantage of the TLT over other methods is represented by the retrograde dilation of the stoma.[10] As far as the comparison between the TLT and OIPs is concerned, the first studies, adopting the usual criteria and the preselection, demonstrated that both kinds of techniques proved equally safe and recommended. These conclusions are open to discussion considering that TLT has completely eliminated most of the risks typical of OIPs, like tracheal damage, ring fractures and bleeding. Many are the studies indicating TLT as the most eligible technique for the most difficult cases.[11-14]

Sixth: There is a frequent underestimation of some complications. To give an example, considering a bruising of the posterior tracheal wall as a small drawback, is not correct, if we consider that between bruising and laceration or perforation there is only pure luck. Indeed, the weight of these complications is much more consistent as it demonstrates that technique has brought the operator closer to a major incident.

Seventh: It is wrong to include in the list of complications some postprocedural events not directly dependent on the type of tracheostomy technique, such as accidental decannulation, which is strictly dependent on the nursing, not on the type of tracheostomy. With a high level of assistance, the frequency of the decannulation is very low. In our unit, for over thirty years, all the patients on controlled ventilation are submitted to supine-prone positioning, that we consider mandatory in every form of respiratory failure, including the cases of neurological patients with normal lungs at the beginning of the treatment. In a thousand patients, thanks to the great dedication of the staff to this procedure, the problem of accidental decannulation has not been felt with any kind of tracheostomy.

Eighth: Every new technique sooner or later, is followed by some variations proposed with the aim of making improvements or to save time through

shortcuts. Under the label of PDT, for instance, are grouped many varieties of the original Ciaglia method (straight dilators instead of curves, different modality of ventilation, and so on), which have their own kind of complications. It is necessary in studies to clearly highlight the adopted variation in order to avoid attributing occurred complications to the original method, with consequent detriment to its reputation, and clinical acceptance.

The same fact has occurred with TLT. A peculiar advantage of our basic method is the possibility of the maintenance of an adequate respiratory support for the whole duration of the procedure, as we have ascertained even in the patients with most severe acute lung injury. Complained episodes of hypercapnia are now and again reported as drawbacks of TLT. Analysing these papers, one discovers that the ventilation catheter is withdrawn before the translaryngeal entering of the cone-cannula, on view to facilitate the subsequent maneuvre of the inversion of the cannula, an issue that does not exist if the needless use of a large cannula, e.g. 9.5 mm ID, is avoided. This procedure is not advisable because it exposes to unacceptable risks of desaturation if an unexpected difficulty, e.g. an accidental decannulation, causes an abnormal prolongation of the procedure.

Ninth: A mere list of complications is usually made without any other characterization except by grouping them by seriousness. This fact considerably limits the power of comparison for the poor value of the information. The necessity to reach a satisfactory reliability of the comparisons demands a deeper insight of the techniques of tracheostomy. Starting from the observation that a tracheostomy is a complex succession of different moments that can be sectioned into three distinct phases (Table 17.1), we adopted this subdivision to obtain a more detailed analysis of the procedure.[15]

In this scheme only the three techniques that we have largely tested have been considered, but this subdivision can be extended to every other method.

For the ST, there is a different definition of the phases but the similarity of the maneuvres is easy detectable. For TLT the third phase has been called inversion because the cannula is already positioned inside the trachea and should only be turned caudally.

Table 17.1: Different phases of tracheostomy

Phase	1	2	3
ST	dissection	trachea opening	cannula insertion
PDT	Needle insertion	dilation	cannula insertion
TLT	Needle insertion	dilation	cannula insertion

We have been using this subdivision for a few years and we have found it undoubtedly useful for the following reasons:
- The description of the technique is more circumstantial.
- The grouping of complications into clearly defined stages allows one to trace their pathogenesis. For example, hemorrhages or tracheal lesions are originated by completely different causes, whether they happen at Phases 1, 2 or 3.
- Risks, difficulties and advantages can have a clear location along the course of the procedure, giving precision and easiness to confrontations.
- The subdivision puts in evidence an important concept: the Phase 1 is similar to every percutaneous method and therefore it is not specific of a particular technique. On the contrary, the Phases 2 and 3 are the distinctive features of each technique and their pros and cons should be the only data to be considered for comparisons.
- In addition, the subdivision does not only point out differences and the similarity between different techniques but also between the variations of the same technique by confronting them phase by phase, as it is shown in the following examples:
  a. Differences between the TLT variations of the cannula inversion (Fig. 17.1).
  b. Differences of the phase 2 of different techniques (Fig. 17.2).
  c. Difference of the phase 3 of different technique (Fig. 17.3).

TLT Phase 3

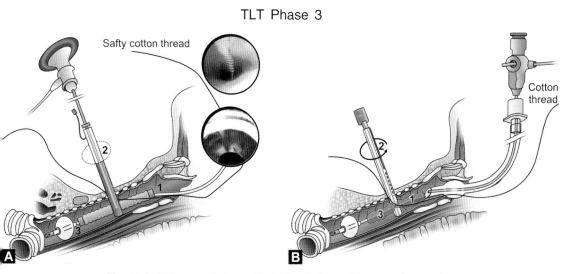

Fig. 17.1: Differences between the TLT variations of the cannula inversion

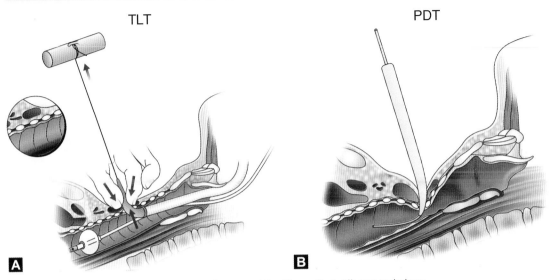

Fig. 17. 2: Difference of the Phase 2 of different technique

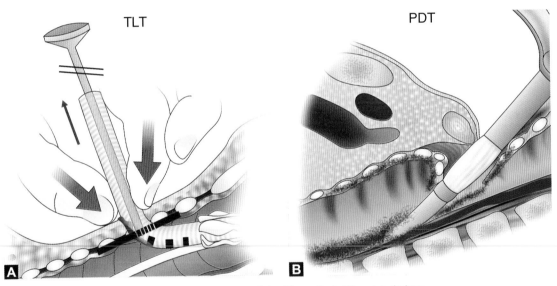

Fig. 17.3: Difference of the Phase 3 of different technique

Tenth: A non-negligible factor in the evaluation of a tracheostomy method is the degree of the hazard of the maneuvres that should not be confounded with the concept of complexity or uncommon procedures.

Criticisms, made by some users about the difficulties of the maneuvres of Phase 3 at the beginning of their experience in the TLT, are the illustrative examples of how a novelty can be seen with mistrust. Actually, the methodology of Phase 3 is easy to learn and ensures the maximum amount of safety because the inversion of the cannula could give way, at the most, to a decannulation. In a patient properly ventilated this is to be taken more as a simple incident, easily remediable by means of the safety thread, than a true complication.

If one examines the corresponding maneuvres of the group of OIP methods, he can note the huge difference in potential risks of their phases of dilation and cannula insertion.

CONCLUSIONS

Tracheostomy is a valuable component in the area of respiratory assistance, but it becomes a substantial cause of the patient's unfavorable outcome if it entails too many severe complications. The main difference among the various techniques is related to the different level of intrinsic, non-operator dependent safety that each technique can provide. Poor intrinsic safety means hazardous procedural steps, many complications and many contraindications, as well as with good operators.

The need of reliable comparisons, so as to permit sounder choices, is evident. Our present study contains some suggestions so as to achieve this objective through a way much more thorough and exacting than that one used, or not used at all, up to now, but certainly much more reliable and effective. Simplistic, misleading comparisons must not be accepted any longer. We have already started to fill in a data base form and we have already noticed the advantage of having precious information available to implement a precise score of difficulties for each patient and for the whole competing series.

There are no valid alternatives for a well-structured comparison, unless one does not want to proceed towards the absolute simplification of the issue with the assumption that tracheostomy, boasting the least number of contraindications, is to be considered superior to all the others.

REFERENCES

1. Ciaglia P, Firsching R, Syniec C. Elective percutaneous dilatational tracheostomy: A new simple bedside procedure; preliminary report. Chest 1985;87:715-9.
2. Ciaglia P. Technique, complications, and improvements in percutaneous dilatational tracheostomy. Chest 1999; 115:1229-30.
3. Pothman W, Tonner PH, Schulte am Esch J. Percutaneous dilatational tracheostomy: Risks and benefits. Intensive Care Med 1997;23:610-12.
4. Fantoni A. La tracheostomia percutanea per dilatazione. Atti XXII Corso aggiornamento in Anestesia e Rianimazione, (1992) In CUEM (ed) Milano, pp 1-14.
5. Hazard P, Jones C, Benitone J. Comparative clinical trial of standard operative tracheostomy with percutaneous tracheostomy. Crit Care Med 1991;19: 1018-24.
6. Friedman Y, Fildes J, Mizock B, et al. Comparison of percutaneous and surgical tracheostomies. Chest 1996; 110:480-5.
7. Porter JM, Ivatury RR. Preferred route of tracheostomy-Percutaneous versus open at the bedside: A randomized, prospective study in the surgical intensive care unit. Am Surgeon 1999;65:142-6.
8. Fantoni A, Ripamonti D, Lesmo A, Zanoni CI. Tracheostomia translaringea. Nuova era? Minerva Anestesiol 1996;62:313-25.
9. Fantoni A, Ripamonti D. A non-derivative, non-surgical tracheostomy: The translaryngeal method. Intensive Care Med 1997;23:386-92.
10. Konopke R, Zimmerman T, Volk A, et al. Prospective evaluation of retrograde percutaneous translaryngeal tracheostomy (Fantoni procedure): Technique and results of the Fantoni tracheostomy in a surgical intensive care unit. Head & Nek 2006;28:355-9.
11. Freeman JW, Katsilerou AK, Tan C, Karnik A, Balchin J. Translaryngeal tracheostomy (TLT): UK clinical experience. Crit Care 1997,1(supp 1): P59.
12. Byhahn C, Lischke V, Westphal K. Translaryngeal tracheostomy in highly unstable patients. Anaesthesia 2000;55:678-82.
13. Milligan KR, McCollum JC. Translaryngeal tracheostomy in high-risk patient. Anaesthesia 2000;55:1132.
14. Sharpe MD, Parnes LS, Drower JW, Harris C. Translaryngeal tracheostomy; experience of 340 cases. Laryngoscope 2003;113:530-6.
15. Fantoni A. Nuovi criteri di comparazione: le fasi della tracheostomia ei dati anatomici essenziali. Minerva Anestesiol 2004;70:445-8.

Chapter 18

Care of Tracheostomy and Principles of Endotracheal Suctioning

Sushil P Ambesh

Since the development of percutaneous tracheostomy, there has been an increase in the number of hospitalized patients with tracheostomy tubes *in situ*, with a subsequent increase in the number of tracheostomized patients in general wards. The management and continued care of trachesotomized patients requires a degree of specialist knowledge. These patients and the attending staff need regular input in the form of tube care, humidification, suction, education, advice and prompt intervention in cases such as tube blockage and dislodgement.

The tracheostomy tube once inserted is secured in place and left to heal for 5-7 days, to allow development of a stable and patent cutaneo-endotracheal tract. The tracheostomy site should be dressed with a sterile gauze piece and secured with a ribbon tie around the neck. The tie should not be too loose or too tight (Fig. 18.1). A tracheostomy is an open wound (whether created by standard surgical approach or by percutaneous approach) therefore strict asepsis and universal precautions should be observed. When dual cannula is used, there is usually no need to change the outer cannula. The inner cannula is changed as and when required. Changing the outer cannula within 5-7 days after placement is potentially dangerous due to risk of collapse or closure of tracheal stoma and

subsequent loss of airway. The only indication of change of outer cannula is when the cuff is damaged or a placement of tube with different size or length is required. If change is necessary then it should be done by a skilled person who is trained in the PDT while keeping the PDT kit and equipments for emergency endotracheal intubation ready.

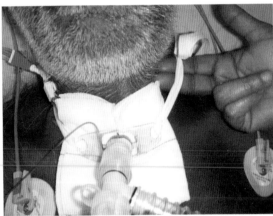

Fig. 18.1: Tracheostomy tube tie (easy insertion of two fingers beneath the tie) and sterile dressings with a half cut gauze piece

Three major factors must be considered during care of a tracheostomized patient:
1. Humidification of inspired gases
2. Mobilization of bronchial secretions and suctioning

3. Patency of the airway and recruitment of collapsed alveoli.

HUMIDIFICATION

The lungs have the largest epithelial surface area of the body in contact with the external environment. In a 24-hours period, an adult man inhales approximately 12,000 to 20,000 litres of air and the airways are continuously exposed to a multitude of particulate matter, pathogens, toxins and noxious gases during respiration that are potentially hazardous. Respiratory mucus acts as a physical barrier, trapping inhaled particles and pathogens, whilst cilia move both the mucus layer and fluid in the underlying pericilliary liquid. The airways, from the nose to the region of the alveoli, are designed to condition the inspired air and to protect the lungs. The upper airways, specially the nose, adequately heat, humidify and filter the inspired air, providing an adequate microambient for an efficient gas exchange at alveoli.[1]

During inspiration, approximately 75% of the water content and heat are provided to the air by nasopharynx, and 25% by the trachea. At the peripheral bronchi, the inspired air reaches 37°C and 100% of relative humidity, which are kept constant up to the alveoli. During exhalation, part of the water content and part of the heat of the expired air are recovered by the mucosa of nasopharynx and trachea. Air filtration also occurs in the conducting airways. The inspired air is completely filtered at the 27th bronchial tree generation. Particles and microorganisms are deposited on the airways walls by impactation and trapped in the mucus blanket lining the surface of the airways. After deposition, mucociliary escalator is activated towards the oropharyngeal region, where the foreign material and cellular debris entrapped in mucus will be removed by swallow or expectoration. Mucociliary clearance efficiency depends on three linked components: ciliated cells, mucus and mucus-cilia interaction. The baseline ciliary activity consists of intact cilia structure in well-organized movements among regions. Decreased mucociliary clearance, once present, may have clinical implications, such as respiratory dysfunction in particular in patients at risk.[2] Colonization and infection results in increased mucus production and increased viscosity of respiratory mucus, which induce prolonged mucociliary clearance. In addition, respiratory mucins may become a place for the carriage and growth of pathogens.

Following formation of tracheostomy the upper airway functions such as filtering, heating and humidification of inspired gases are bypassed. Therefore, the inspired air may have a significant humidity deficit which may lead to pathological changes in the airway such as mucosal damage, loss of mucociliary transport, impaired surfactant activity and thickening of airway secretions.[3,4] The thickened mucous plug may provide loci for lower respiratory tract infections. Dry gases can cause bronchoconstriction, further compromising respiratory function. Though there is no agreement about the minimum humidity necessary to prevent pathological changes, the importance of humidifying and heating the inspired gases can not be overemphasized. It is absolutely essential that adequate humidity be provided to keep the airway moist. The patient must be properly hydrated with oral or IV fluids to permit the mucosal surface to remain moist and to ensure that the viscid secretions remain atop the cilia. This will make the secretions thinner and more mobile.

Inspired gases conditioning can be provided by 2 distinct mechanisms: a heated humidifying system or a heated moisture exchanger also known as artificial nose.

Heat and Moisture Exchanger (HME) or Artificial Nose

The HME conserves the exhaled water and heat, and returns them to the patient in the inspired gas.

The HMEs are also known as a condenser humidifier, artificial nose, Swedish nose, vapor condenser, nose humidifier, passive humidifier or regenerative humidifier (Fig. 18.2). When combined with a filter for bacteria and viruses, it is called a heat and moisture exchanging filter (HMEF). HMEs are disposable devices and vary in size and shape. Each device has a female connection port (15 mm) at the patient end and a male port (15 mm) at the machine end. Most of HMEs contain a port to attach the gas sampling line for a respiratory gas monitor. The HMEs are two types: the hydrophobic or hygroscopic. The hydrophobic HMEs have a hydrophobic membrane that is pleated to increase the surface area. It provides moderately good inspired humidity; however, the performance may be impaired by high ambient temperature. They allow the passage of water vapur but not liquid water and effectively prevent passage of hepatitis C virus on usual ventilatory pressures.[5-7] The HMEs are easy to use, small light weight, simple in design, silent in operation and inexpensive.

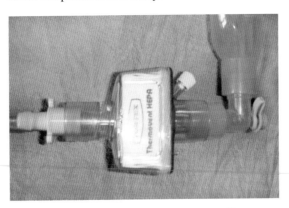

Fig. 18.2: Heat and moisture exchange filter
(SIMS Portex, UK)

The devices do not require water, external source for heating, temperature monitor or alarms. These are quite safe and there is no danger of overhydration, hyperthermia, burns of respiratory mucosa and electric shock. However, the HMEs have some disadvantages. HMEs provide limited humidity, and insignificant contribution in temperature preservation where heated humidifiers are more effective. It also increases work of breathing during both inspiration and expiration. In addition, turbulent airflow during mechanical ventilation decreases inspired air water content and may induce tracheal trauma.

Humidifiers/water Vaporizers

The humidifiers are two types: heated or unheated. Unheated humidifiers are bubble through and can not deliver moisture more than 9 mg H_2O/litre and are of limited value for a tracheostomized patient on ventilator. Heated humidifiers incorporate a device to warm the water in humidifier. The heat may be supplied by heating rods immersed in the water or a plate at the bottom of the humidification chamber. The temperature of the water is regulated by a thermostat that may be servo-controlled or non-servo-controlled. Most heated humidifiers measure the gas temperature at the patient end of the breathing system. There are temperature sensors in the water reservoir or in contact with the heater plate to activate alarms and shut off power source of heater when necessary. If used in the circle system, a heated humidifier is placed in the inspiratory limb downstream of the unidirectional valve by using an accessory breathing tube. If a filter is used in the breathing system then it must be placed upstream of the humidifier to prevent it from becoming clogged.

Most heated humidifiers are capable of delivering saturated gas at or above the body temperature at variable flow rates. They are very effective and may be used for controlled as well as spontaneous respiration in tracheostomized patients. The main disadvantages of these humidifiers are: bulky and complex structure. These devices involve high maintenance cost and electrical hazards. They also require repeated filling, draining, sterilization of reservoir. There are risk of over-hydration, water aspiration, thermal injuries, monitoring interference and infection.

MOBILIZATION OF BRONCHIAL SECRETIONS

Acute illness impairs mucociliary clearance in stable patients with no airway manipulation.[8] Smoking and acute illness further markedly affects mucociliary clearance. Several drugs used in the ICU patients may affect the overall mucociliary clearance. Furosemide, a potent diuretic drug, has been associated with reduced mucociliary transport in patients under mechanical ventilation after 2 hours of drug administration.[9] The association of furosemide and hypovolemia produces a marked reduction in tracheal transepithelial potential difference, a potential factor for mucociliary clearance dysfunction. Alpha and beta adrenergic receptor drugs increase ciliary beating with dose-dependent effect. Benzodiazepines, narcotics, anesthesia are known to affect cough and ciliary activity, and also cause mucus accumulation.

Difficulty in mucus transport by cilia or cough and mucus accumulation in the airways may lead to mucus accumulation, airway obstruction, bacterial colonization and respiratory infection, which may ultimately contribute to increased morbidity and mortality in critically ill patients. Many of the nursing skills employed are aimed at the mobilization of pulmonary secretions. Frequent turning, encouragement of deep breathing, and ambulation are important in the prevention of pulmonary complications. Regular chest physiotherapy and postural drainage are both very effective in the mobilization of secretions and should be used routinely during the postoperative period. Manual ventilation (bagging) along with tracheal instillation of normal saline may also aid in the mobilization of secretions.

ENDOTRACHEAL SUCTIONING

Patients ventilated through ET tube or tracheostomy tube are unable to clear secretions effectively as glottic closure is compromised and normal mucociliary function is impaired.[10] Inadequately

humidified inspired gas and the presence of the tracheal tube may cause irritation of the airways with a resulting increase in secretion production.[11] Therefore, all patients with an artificial airway require endotracheal suctioning to remove secretions and prevent airway obstruction in order to maintain an optimal level of ventilation.[12]

Suctioning is an uncomfortable procedure and is usually a frightening one for an awake patient. It is a procedure where both psychological and physiological defensive reflexes will come into play for the protection of the airway. Although considered essential to prevent airway obstruction from accumulation of secretions, it is recognized that severe adverse events may result from suctioning. These include hypoxia, cardiac dysrrhythmias,[13,14] increased intracranial pressure,[15] bacteremia,[10] pneumothorax, mucosal trauma,[16] atelectasis,[17] loss of ciliary function[10] and negative pressure pulmonary edema.[18] Endotracheal suctioning has also been shown to cause pain and discomfort.[19] It is, therefore, important to monitor patients carefully at all times during suctioning. Some of the above complications may be due to vagal nerve stimulation, coughing or catheter trauma and others may be directly related to the physical effects of suctioning on the lungs. Atelectasis has been attributed to the aspiration of intrapulmonic gas,[20] mucosal edema,[17] or bronchial obstruction as a result of mucosal trauma.[21]

Disconnection from the ventilator during open ET suctioning results in a decrease in airway pressure with loss of lung volume, and further lung volume loss occurs with the application of a negative pressure during suctioning.[22] Maggiore et al, found that endexpiratory lung volume decreased during ET suctioning, regardless of the suctioning technique performed: open suction, through swivel adaptor or through a closed suction system. The extent of lung volume loss during suctioning appears to be directly related to the size of the catheter in relation to the ETT size.[23,24] Therefore, it is important that the catheter used for suctioning should not be so large that it traumatises or occludes the airway, which would lead to greater negative pressure accumulation[23] and lung volume loss[24] but should be large enough to effectively suction thick secretions. Doubling the ETT internal diameter gives an indication of which FG catheter size to use for efficacy and safety (for example, with a 3.5 mm ID ETT, a size 6 or 7 FG catheter should be used).

It has been suggested that ET suctioning causes a decrease in airway resistance, by the removal of pulmonary secretions.[25] However, Morrow et al[24] showed that ET suctioning did not have a significant effect on dynamic airway resistance in 78 ventilated pediatric patients. Guglielminotti et al[12] also found that resistance did not decrease below presuction levels after an initial increase related to transient bronchoconstriction. Airway resistance may decrease significantly if large amounts of mucus are removed from the airways during suctioning.

Indications for Suctioning

Suctioning should never be considered routine but should be based upon several observations: audible secretions, coughing, desaturation, a rise in peak inspiratory pressure, increased airway resistance, increased work of breathing, decrease dynamic compliance, decreased tidal volume delivery during pressure-limited ventilation, increasing patient apprehension, evidence of atelectasis on chest X-ray or rhonchi heard by auscultation. Both sides of the chest should be routinely auscultated with a stethoscope. If patients are ventilated using machines with displayed flow-volume loops, a saw-toothed pattern may indicate the presence of secretions in the ETT. Patients receiving high frequency oscillatory ventilation should be observed with regard to the amount of the chest wall oscillation – if this changes it may indicate the presence of secretions. Routine suctioning may actually stimulate production of airway secretions and can be associated with more adverse effects.

In order to minimize the recurrent derecruitment and subsequent rerecruitment on reconnection to the ventilator caused by suctioning, which may exacerbate lung injury;[22] ET suctioning should be kept to a minimum. Negative pressure in the lungs produced during suctioning would only occur while air was flowing through the suction catheter. As soon as secretions are drawn into the catheter, the pressure in the lungs would return to that of the atmosphere.[26] Therefore, suctioning in the absence of secretions may exacerbate lung volume loss and no clear benefit of a routine regimen of ET suctioning has been demonstrated. ET suctioning should be performed only when clinically indicated in order to maximise secretion removal; and minimise the complications, pain and discomfort to the patient. Exceptions to this may include patients receiving muscle relaxants who will not be able to cough.

Vacuum Pressure

There is still no good evidence supporting a maximum safe, and effective suction level but Morrow et al[23] suggested that suction pressures up to 360 mm Hg measured at the vacuum source were more effective in removing secretions than using vacuum pressures of approximately 200 mm Hg. These suction pressures are higher than that recommended by some authors[27,28] but are within the range used in clinical practice worldwide.[29] Until clear evidence is available, it is suggested that practitioners use the lowest pressure that effectively removes the secretions, with the least adverse clinical reaction. Suction pressures should be < 400 mm Hg.

Sterility

Although the introduction of a catheter into the ETT presents the opportunity for introducing infection, it does not appear to be necessary to use a sterile suctioning technique. In a randomized controlled trial of 486 intubated children and infants, it was found that reusing a disposable suction catheter in the same patient over a 24-hour period did not affect the incidence of pneumonia.[30]

Suctioning Technique

When you have gathered all necessary equipments, take time to reassure and explain the procedure to your patient. The communication with a tracheostomized patient is quite difficult. Give the patient a pencil and paper, or word your questions so that the patient can indicate "Yes" or "No" by nodding his/her head or blinking his/her eyes. Always remember to preoxygenate your patient before the suction procedure and to constantly observe for clinical signs that may indicate hypoxia.

In an attempt to minimize or prevent hypoxia, it has been recommended that patients should receive increased inspired oxygen levels prior to suctioning.[28,31] Pritchard et al,[32] in a systematic *Cochrane* review, showed that preoxygenation decreased hypoxaemia at the time of suctioning, but other clinically important outcomes, including the adverse effects of hyperoxia, were not known. Considering the short-term effects in reducing ET-suctioning induced hypoxia, it is recommended that patients be given increased FiO_2 for a brief period (one minute) prior to suctioning. There is no high-level evidence to support an appropriate level of preoxygenation, but it is suggested that the degree of increase in inspired oxygen may be determined by the individual's response to general handling and ET suctioning. Hyperoxia is associated with oxygen free-radical damage, which is associated with major morbidity,[33] and may also cause absorption atelectasis.[34] It is, therefore, essential to return the FiO_2 to pre-suctioning levels as soon as the oxygen saturation has stabilised in order to prevent the adverse effects of hyperoxia. Increasing the duration of suction application has been shown to significantly increase the amount of negative pressure within a lung model and exacerbate hypoxia.[35] There is currently no strong

evidence supporting an appropriate duration of suctioning, but times from 5 to 15 seconds have been advocated.[31,36,37]

The catheter should only be passed to just beyond the distal tip of the tracheal tube. There are no benefits to performing deep suctioning and there is an increased risk of direct trauma, vagal nerve stimulation and ciliary disfunction[1] with deep rather than shallow suctioning.[38]

Instillation of isotonic saline (sodium chloride) has been a widespread practice for many years, under the impression that the fluid aided in the removal of pulmonary secretions by lubricating the catheter, eliciting a cough and diluting secretions. However, mucus and water in bulk form are immiscible and maintain their separate phases even after vigorous shaking.[39] Thus, the function of saline as a secretion dilutant is doubtful. Several studies have now reported the adverse effect of saline instillation on arterial oxygenation.[40-42] Instillation of normal saline in conjunction with ET suctioning also results in additional dispersion of contaminated adherent material in the lower respiratory tract, with the subsequent increased risk of nosocomial infection.[43] In order to ensure that pulmonary secretions are easily manageable with suctioning, it is essential to ensure adequate humidification of inspired gas.[44]

Closed versus Open Suctioning

A closed (in-line) suction catheter utilizes an enclosed transparent, flexible plastic sleeve that is attached to a specially designed T-piece adapter, which is left in place adjacent to the tracheal tube. The adapter contains a sealing assembly to prevent gas leaks around the catheter and to remove secretions from its external surface as it is drawn back into the sheath. At the other end there is a manual vacuum control and connection for the suction tubing. It may be possible to lock the suction control valve in the OFF position. An irrigation port may be present at either end for tracheal lavage with the catheter inserted or for rinsing the catheter. It has been suggested that use of a closed-suction system may prevent ET suctioning induced hypoxia and decreases in lung volume in pediatric[45] and adult[46] patients and may reduce the rate of ventilator associated pneumonia[47] Closed-system suctioning can be performed through an adaptor inserted at the ETT-ventilator circuitry interface. When not in use the catheter rests in withdrawn position just outside the airway (Fig. 18.3).[48]

Another potential benefit of using closed-system suctioning may be the limitation of aerosolisation of infectious mucus particles; thereby preventing the spread of infection between patients and from patients to staff.[49] However, there are some drawbacks of closed-system suctioning and that include the risk of producing high negative pressures [50] if the amount of air suctioned exceeds the gas flow delivered to the patient by the ventilator;[51] reduced efficiency in clearing thick secretions from the airways;[52] and the high financial cost of the system which has to be replaced daily in order to avoid microbial lower respiratory tract colonization.[43] Woodgate and Flenady[53] concluded from a systematic review that there was insufficient evidence to decide between ET suctioning with or without disconnection, despite some potential short-term benefits associated with closed-system suctioning.

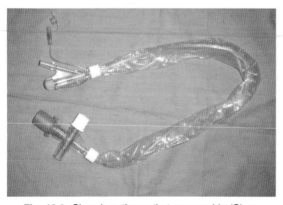

Fig. 18.3: Closed suction catheter assembly (Sims, Portex, UK)

The risk of serious side-effects increases with the severity of the patients' disease. The higher the PEEP level needed, the greater the risk of severe heart/lung interactions, especially loss of end expiratory lung volume and hypoxemia, and already at disconnection of the ventilator.[54]

It is clear that suctioning should only be performed on strict indications such as bubbling secretions in the trachea or increasing airway resistance. To suction a patient just because an hour has passed is an insufficient reason, but to wait until there are secretions evident in the bronchial tree may not be appropriate. Research has been focused on the side-effects, rather than the effectiveness of secretion removal. The closed system was introduced in the early eighties as it enables ventilation during suctioning, avoiding disconnection from the ventilator. Thus, the side effects of the closed suction system have been thoroughly evaluated in contrast to suction efficacy, where only qualitative or semi-quantitative reports are available. However, in one recent bench study, closed system suctioning was shown to be about five times less effective than open suctioning.[55] These findings have also recently been confirmed in a patient study.[56] Resistance to flow through the endotracheal tube, with the inserted suction catheter, is high. This increased resistance to flow from ambient air towards the suction catheter tip in the trachea is larger than the resistance from the lungs, because the cross-sectional area of the trachea is about 250 mm^2 and the area between the inner surface of a 7 mm inner diameter (ID) endotracheal tube and a 12 Fr suction catheter (4 mm outer diameter) is 38–13 mm^2 = 25 mm^2. Thus, during open suctioning, gas is aspirated from the lungs rather than from room air. During closed system suctioning, with normal trigger sensitivity, sub-atmospheric lung pressures are avoided as the ventilator interpret the suction flow as a breathing demand, responding by delivering a tidal volume, which helps overcome the resistance of the endotracheal tube and feeds the suction catheter with gas, minimising suction from the airway below the suction catheter tip. The triggered inspiratory gas inflow can be seen to push secretions away from the catheter tip[55] and there is less likelihood of movement of the secretions from the lungs.

Conversely, during open suctioning, gas aspirated from the lung will probably facilitate the movement of secretions towards the suction catheter. Finally, the rapid change in lung volume following disconnection of the ventilator for open suctioning may initiate a cough, moving secretions towards the suction catheter. The less side-effects of closed system suctioning are highly dependent on how the suctioning procedure is handled. The use of large suction catheters, very high vacuum levels or disadvantageous ventilator settings can result in similar or worse side-effects than an open suctioning procedure.[57] There is a possibility to create a completely closed system if the resistance in the tube cannot be overcome by the ventilator, when the interior surface is lined with thick secretions and/or a very thick catheter is used, and/or the trigger function of the ventilator is deactivated. In such a situation the suctioning flow will empty the lungs rapidly and if the suctioning procedure has a sufficient duration the pressure in the lungs will be the same as the vacuum level in the suctioning system. This can lead to damage on both patient and ventilator.

Using a vacuum level of -50 kPa (-375 mm Hg, -500 cm H_2O), the initial suction flow through a 12 Fr (X 4.0 mm) catheter, when the switch is opened, is around 18 l/min for some seconds. The duration of this "high flow period" depends on the size of the suction bottle and will be shorter with a small one than a large one. The flow reaches a steady state at 13 l/min. The corresponding values for a 14 Fr (X 4.6 mm) catheter are 43 and 23 l/min.[57] It is noteworthy that changing catheter diameter with 0.6 mm results in a large increase in flow, especially the initial flow. When closed system suctioning is started with a 14 Fr catheter, 670 ml is suctioned during the first second and if the trigger function of the ventilator is deactivated or secretions inside the tube prevents ventilation during suctioning, this volume will be removed from the lungs.

When handled correctly, closed system suctioning has less side-effects than open suctioning, but the suctioning procedure may have to be repeated several times in order to reach the same degree of secretion removal as during an open suctioning procedure.[56,57] Closed system suctioning during continuous positive pressure ventilation with a moderate pressure level could be a tolerable compromise to optimise efficiency and side-effects.[55] Another alternative is to convert to open suctioning combined with a subsequent recruitment manoeuvre.[58]

Recruitment of Collapsed Alveoli

Recruitment maneuvres have been proposed as a means of reversing suctioning induced lung volume loss by recruiting atelectatic regions of the lung, thereby improving arterial oxygenation.[29,59] A recruitment maneuvre refers to the application of a sustained inflation pressure to the lungs for a specified duration, in order to return the lung to normal volumes and distribution of air. However, because clinical trials have shown a variable response to recruitment maneuvres (including no effect and adverse reactions) more information regarding safety, efficacy, indications, and technique is needed from clinical studies before recruitment maneuvres can be recommended as part of the standard management of ventilated patients.[60,61]

Monitoring of Tube Cuff Pressure

Most patients who undergo tracheostomy require cuffed tracheostomy tube in order to prevent aspiration and to facilitate controlled ventilation. The balloon of the artificial airway may also impose additional risks for tracheal complications such as local distension, hypoperfusion and decreased ciliary activity. Tracheostomy tube cuff requires monitoring to maintain pressures in the range of 20-25 mm Hg (at end-expiration).[62] High cuff pressures above 30 mmHg may jeopardize capillary perfusion and may result in mucosal ischemia and tracheal stenosis. Low cuff pressures below 18 mm Hg may cause development of longitudinal folds in tracheal cuff, promoting microaspiration of secretions collected above the cuff and increase the risk of nosocomial pneumonia. The pressure should be measured and adjusted approximately 10 minutes after the tube has been inserted. This delay is necessary to allow for softening of the cuff material at body temperature and for the patient to become settled, because the volume necessary for occlusion will vary with muscle tone. Following adjustment of cuff pressure a check should be made to ensure that there is no leak at peak airway pressure. The endotracheal cuff pressures should be monitored at least once per change of nursing shift and after each manipulation of tracheostomy tube. It has been suggested to periodically deflate the cuff to allow mucosal perfusion at the site of tracheal cuff and to improve clearance of secretions accumulated around the cuff; however, there is no evidence that support this practice. It is important to maintain the tracheal tube in central position and avoid dragging or traction on it to avoid erosion of tracheal mucosa by tip of the tube.

Key Major Recommendations

Following formation of tracheostomy the upper airway functions such as filtering, heating and humidification of inspired gases are bypassed. The importance of humidifying and heating the inspired gases can not be overemphasized and it is absolutely essential that adequate humidity be provided to keep the airway moist. ET suctioning, although necessary to maintain patency of the airways, is not a benign procedure. All staff performing the procedure should be aware of the positive and negative effects of ET suctioning as well as methods to prevent or minimise the known complications of the procedure.

Therefore, it is essential to remember several things when suctioning a patient:

1. A tracheostomy is an open wound (whether created by standard surgical approach or by percutaneous approach) therefore strict asepsis and universal precautions should be observed. Wash your hands with soap and water or antimicrobial solutions; put on sterile gloves.

2. Explanation the procedure and reassure the patient as it is known to decrease the patient's anxiety and fears.

3. Select a disposable sterile suction catheter according to the size of tracheostomy tube. The outer diameter of the suction catheter should not exceed 50% of the ID of the lumen being suctioned. A suction catheter of greater diameter could lead to obstruction to the air flow around the catheter during the procedure. The smallest catheter necessary to remove the secretions should be selected. It may be helpful to wrap the catheter around the glove hand to reduce the risk of contamination.

4. Set the negative pressure by occluding the suction tubing and adjusting the regulator while observing the gauge. The negative pressure for suctioning the trachea should be no greater than 70-150 mm Hg (50-150 cm H_2O, 9.3 to 20 kPa) in adults and 60-80 mm Hg in infants.

5. Lubricate tip of catheter by dipping tip in sterile saline or by rolling in sterile water-soluble lubricant prior to insertion. The catheter should be inserted with a smooth, gentle motion, without force or without applying any negative pressure. The catheter should be passed just beyond the end of tracheal tube to avoid tracheal mucosa injury.

6. Partial occlusion of the airway by the suction catheter, combined with aspiration of air from the lung, can result in severe hypoxia, cardiac arrhythmia, and even cardiac arrest. Suctioning procedures should be kept for a minimum and must never exceed 15 seconds even if no visible signs of stress are noted.

7. The upper airway is lined with delicate tissue and care must be taken to avoid damage to these tissues during suctioning. For this reason, suction is applied only intermittently and with catheter rotation to avoid trauma to the mucosal walls of the trachea and bronchi.

8. Apply the suction during withdrawal of catheter in order to decrease the volume of air removed from the lungs and decrease the hypoxic effect and trauma to the airway. Rotate the catheter gently between your thumb and forefinger during withdrawal.

9. Reoxygenate the patient after withdrawal of the catheter and check adequate tidal volume is delivered.

10. Check the vitals and stability of hemodynamics before leaving the patient side.

Home Care of Tracheostomized Patients

A Eurovent study[63] showed that there were more than 21000 patients receiving home ventilation in Europe for their neuromuscular disorders (1/3), parenchymal lung disease (1/3) and chest wall disorders (1/3). About 13% patients had tracheostomy ventilation and around 10% (>2000) were in the pediatric age group. Life in hospital is an unsuitable environment for the developing child and an inappropriate use of resources. In 1999, a cross sectional survey of 141 children from the United Kingdom reported that 24% were ventilated by tracheostomy, and 68% were cared for at home.[64] Patients can be treated in their homes and live "normal" lives.

Home care of children with tracheostomy is a special challenge. Adequate care involves the family and a multidisciplinary team of caregivers. Communication with community based health caregivers must start as soon as possible. A key role of the hospital team is teaching and training of children, parents and community based health caregivers. Theoretical and practical courses in tracheostomy care and the use of ventilators should be arranged regularly or on request to train parents and community based caregivers. The parents are taught stoma care and correct suction technique for a week. At first the parents observe the procedure, later they are taught to perform a canula change under supervision. The parents must perform the procedure several times before the child is discharged to home care. The intensive care nurse from the "home ventilator" team visits during the first few canulas change at home. The parents are trained in various aspects of their child care, such as inhalation therapy and maintenance of the technical medical equipment. Parents are also trained to perform basic life support with the use of a ventilation bag and oxygen.

Use of silicone tracheostomy canulas are preferred in children as these are soft and less irritative than canulas made of plastic or metal. Children find it easier to eat and swallow, and it is easier to change the canula. Though the silicone canula is expensive, but it can be cleaned and boiled at home and reused by the same child. A child usually needs 3 or 4 canulas per year. The canulas can be used as long as they are undamaged, and the size requirement stays the same.

It is important that all personnel must fulfill a procedure checklist and verified by a tutor, before they start working with the child. The intensive care nurse should visit the patients at home on a regular basis and should be available for telephone consultations. The parents should be free to visit hospital if need be. All children should have a named consultant in the hospital and a general practitioner or family doctor in the community. An essential part of the care plan is an individual booklet with procedures and practical information. This booklet follows the patient and should be available at all times for the parents and caregivers.

REFERENCES

1. Nakagawa NK, Macchione M, Petrolino HMS, Guimaraes ET, King M, Saldiva PHN, Lorenzi-Filho G. Effects of a heat and moisture exchanger and a heated humidifier on respiratory mucus in patients undergoing mechanical ventilation. Crit Care Med 2000;28:312-7.

2. Boucher RC. New concepts of the pathogenesis of cystic fibrosis lung disease. Eur Respir J 2004;23:146-58.

3. Branson R, Campbell R, Davis K, et al. Anaesthesia circuits, humidity output, and mucociliary structure and function. Anaesth Intens Care 1998;26:178-83.

4. Williams R, Rankin N, Smith T, et al. Relationship between the humidity and temperature of inspired gas and the function of airway mucosa. Crit Care Med 1996;24:1920-9.

5. Hedley RM, Allt-Graham J. A comparison of the filtration properties of heat and moisture exchangers. Anaesthesia 1992;47:414-20.

6. Lee MG, Ford JL, Hunt PB, et al. Bacterial retention properties of heat and moisture exchange filters. Br J Anaesth 1992;69:522-5.

7. Lloyd G, Howells J, Liddle C, et al. Barriers to hepatitis C transmission within breathing systems:Efficacy of pleated hydrophobic filter. Anaesth Intens Care 1997;25:325-38.

8. Nakagawa NK, Franchini ML, Driusso P, Oliveira LR, Saldiva PHN, Lorenzi-Filho G. Mucociliary clearance is impaired in acutely ill patients. Chest 2005;128:2772-7.

9. Kondo CS, Macchione M, Nakagawa NK, Carvalho CRR, King M, Saldiva PHN, Lorenz-Filho G. Effects of intravenous furosemide on mucociliary transport and rheological properties of patients under mechanical ventilation. Crti Care 2002;6:81-7.

10. Bailey C, Kattwinkel J, Teja K, Buckley T. Shallow versus deep endotracheal suctioning in young rabbits: Pathological effects on the tracheobronchial wall. Pediatrics 1988;82:746-51.

11. Fisher BJ, Carlo WA, Doershuk CF. in Scarpelli EM (ED) Pulmonary Physiology: Fetus, Newborn, Child, Adolescent. Second Edition, Lea & Febiger 1990; Philadelphia, USA pp 422-8.

12. Guglielminotti J, Desmonts J, Dureuil B. Effects of tracheal suctioning on respiratory resistances in mechanically ventilated patients. Chest 1998;113:1335-8.

13. Kohlhauser C, Bernert G, Hermon M, Popow C, Seidl R, Pollak A. Effects of endotracheal suctioning in high – frequency oscillatory and conventionally ventilated low birth weight neonates on cerebral hemodynamics observed by near infrared spectroscopy (NIRS). Pediatr. Pulmonol 2000;29:270-5.

14. Simbruner G, Coradello H, Foder M, Havelec L, Lubec G, Pollak A. Effect of tracheal suction on oxygenation, circulation, and lung mechanics in newborn infants. Arch Dis Child 1981;56:326-30.

15. Kerr ME, Weber BB, Sereika SM, Darby J, Marion DW, Orndoff PA. Effect of endotracheal suctioning on cerebral oxygenation in traumatic brain – injured patients. Crit Care Med 1999;27:2776-81.

16. Loubser MD, Mahoney PJ, Milligan DW. Hazards of routine endotracheal suction in the neonatal unit. Lancet 1989;1(8652):1444-5.

17. Boothroyd AE, Murthy BVS, Darbyshire A, Petros AJ. Endotracheal suctioning causes right upper lobe collapse in intubated children. Acta Paediatr 1996;85:1422-5.

18. Pang WW, Chang DP, Lin CH et al. Negative pressure pulmonary oedema induced by direct suctioning of endotracheal tube adapter. Can J Anaesth 1998;45:785-8.

19. Simons SH, van Dijk M, Anand KS, Roofthooft D, van Lingen RA, Tibboel D. Do we still hurt newborn babies? A prospective study of procedural pain and analgesia in neonates. Arch Pediatr Adolesc Med 2003;157:1058-64.

20. Ehrhart IC, Hofman WF, Loveland SR. Effects of endotracheal suction versus apnea during interruption of intermittent or continuous positive pressure ventilation. Crit Care Med 1981;9:464-8.

21. Nagaraj HS, Fellows R, Shott R, Yacoub U. Recurrent lobar atelectasis due to acquired bronchial stenosis in neonates. J Pediatr Surg 1980;15:411-5.

22. Maggiore SM, Lellouche F, Pigeot J, et al. Prevention of Endotracheal Suctioning-induced Alveolar Derecruitment in Acute Lung Injury. Am J Respir Crit Care Med 2003;167:1215-24.

23. Morrow B, Futter M, Argent A. Endotracheal suctioning: From principles to practice. Int Care Med 2004;30:1167-74.

24. Morrow B, Futter M, Argent A. Effect of endotracheal suction on lung dynamics in mechanically ventilated paediatric patients. Aust J Physiother 2006;52:121-6.

25. Fox WW, Schwartz JG, Shaffer TH. Pulmonary physiotherapy in neonates: Physiologic changes and respiratory management. J Pediatrics 1978;92:977-81.

26. Rosen M, Hillard EK. The effects of negative pressure during tracheal suction. Anesthesia and Analgesia Current Researches 1962;41:50-7.

27. Kacmarek RM, Stoller JK. Principles of Respiratory Care. *In* Shoemaker WC, Ayres SM, Grenvik A, Holbrook P (Eds.). Textbook of Critical Care. Third Edition. USA, WB Saunders Company 1995; p. 695.

28. Hodge D. Endotracheal suctioning and the infant: A nursing care protocol to decrease complications. Neonatal Network 1991;9:7-15.

29. Dyhr T, Bonde J, Larsson A. Lung recruitment manoeuvres are effective in regaining lung volume and oxygenation after open endotracheal suctioning in acute respiratory distress syndrome. Critical Care 2003;7: 55-62.

30. Scoble MK, Copnell B, Taylor A, Kinney S, Shann F. Effect of reusing suction catheters on the occurrence of pneumonia in children. Heart & Lung 2001;30:225-33.

31. Branson RD, Campbell RS, Chatburn RL, Covington JC. AARC Clinical Practice Guideline: Endotracheal suctioning of mechanically ventilated adults and children with artificial airways. Respir Care 1993;38:500-04.

32. Pritchard M, Flenady V, Woodgate P. Preoxygenation for tracheal suctioning in intubated, ventilated newborn infants (Cochrane Review). In: *The Cochrane Library*, 2003; Issue 3. Oxford: Update Software.

33. Inder TE, Volpe JJ. Mechanisms of perinatal brain injury. Semin Neonatol 2000;5(1):3-16.

34. Rothen HU, Sporre B, Engberg G, Wegenius G, Hogman M, Hedenstierna G. Influence of gas composition on recurrence of atelectasis after a reexpansion maneuver during general anesthesia. Anesthesiology 1995;82: 832-42.

35. Brandstater B, Muallem M. Atelectasis Following Tracheal Suction in Infants. Anesthesiology 1969; 31:468-73.

36. Young J. To help or hinder: Endotracheal suction and the intubated neonate. Journal of Neonatal Nursing 1995; 1:23-8.

37. Runton N. Suctioning artificial airways in children: Appropriate technique. Paediatric Nursing 1992;18: 115-8.

38. Youngmee A, Yonghoon J. The effects of the shallow and the deep endotracheal suctioning on oxygen saturation and heart rate in high-risk infants. International Journal of Nursing Studies 2003;40: 97-104.

39. Demers RR, Saklad M. Minimizing the harmful effects of mechanical aspiration: Aspects of respiratory care. Heart Lung 1973;2:542-5.

40. Ridling DA, Martin LD, Bratton SL. Endotracheal Suctioning With or Without Instillation of Isotonic Sodium Chloride Solution in Critically Ill Children. Am J Crit Care 2003;12:212-9.

41. Kinloch D. Instillation of normal saline during endotracheal suctioning: Effects on mixed venous oxygen saturation. Am J Crit Care 1999;8:231-40.

42. Ackerman MH, Mick DJ. Instillation of normal saline before suctioning in patients with pulmonary infections: A prospective randomised controlled trial. Am J Crit Care 1998;7:261-6.

43. Freytag CC, Thies FL, König W, Welte T. Prolonged application of closed in-line suction catheters increases microbial colonisation of the lower respiratory tract and bacterial growth on catheter surface. Infection 2003; 31:31-7.

44. Branson RD, Campbell RS, Chatburn RL, Covington JC. AARC Clinical Practice Guideline: Humidification during mechanical ventilation. Respir Care 1992;37:887-90.

45. Choong K, Chatrkaw P, Frndova H, Cox PN. Comparison of loss in lung volume with open versus in-line catheter endotracheal suctioning. Pediatr Crit Care Med 2003;4:69-73.

46. Cereda M, Villa F, Colombo E, Greco G, Nacoti M, Pesenti A. Closed system endotracheal suctioning maintains lung volume during volume-controlled mechanical ventilation. Int Care Med 2001;27:648-54.

47. Combes P, Fauvage B, Oleyer C. Nosocomial pneumonia in mechanically ventilated patients, a prospective randomized evaluation of the Stericath closed suctioning system. Int Care Med 2000;26:878-82.

48. Taggart JA, Dorinsky NL, Sheahan JS. Airway pressures during closed system suctioning. Heart Lung 1988;17: 536-42.

49. Cobley M, Atkins M, Jones FL. Environmental contamination during tracheal suction: A comparison of disposable conventional catheters with a multiple-use closed system device. Anaesthesia 1991;46:957-61.

50. Stenqvist O, Lindgren S, Karason S, Söndergaard S, Lundin S. Warning! Suctioning. A lung model evaluation of closed suctioning systems. Acta Anaesthesiologica Scandinavica 2001;45:167-72.

51. Strindlund M. Personal communication via letter from General Manager, Siemans Medical Solutions; 2002.

52. Lindgren S, Almgren B, Högman M, et al. Effectiveness and side effects of closed and open suctioning: An experimental evaluation. Int Care Med 2004;31:1630-37.

53. Woodgate PG, Flenady V. Tracheal suctioning without disconnection in intubated ventilated neonates (Cochrane Review). In: *The Cochrane Library, 2003;* Issue 3. Oxford: Update Software.

54. Maggiore SM, Lellouche F, Pigeot J, Taille S, Deye N, Durrmeyer X, Richard J-C, Mancebo J, Lemaire F, Brochard L: Prevention of Endotracheal Suctioning-induced Alveolar Derecruitment in Acute Lung Injury. Am J Respir Crit Care Med 2003;167:1215-24.

55. Lindgren S, Almgren B, Hogman M, Lethvall S, Houltz E, Lundin S, Stenqvist O: Effectiveness and side effects of closed and open suctioning: An experimental evaluation. Intensive Care Med 2004;30:1630-7.

56. Lasocki S, Lu Q, Sartorius A, Fouillat D, Remerand F, Rouby JJ: Open and Closed-circuit Endotracheal Suctioning in Acute Lung Injury: Efficiency and Effects on Gas Exchange. Anesthesiology 2006;104:39-47.

57. Stenqvist O, Lindgren S, Karason S, Sondergaard S, Lundin S: Warning! Suctioning. A lung model evaluation of closed suctioning systems. Acta Anaesthesiol Scand 2001, 45:167-72.

58. Dyhr T, Bonde J, Larsson A: Lung recruitment manoeuvres are effective in regaining lung volume and oxygenation after open endotracheal suctioning in acute respiratory distress syndrome. Crit Care 2003;7:55-62.

59. Matthews BD, Noviski N. Management of oxygenation in pediatric acute hypoxemic respiratory failure. Ped Pulmonol 2001;32:459-70.

60. ARDS Clinical trials Network; National Heart, Lung and Blood Institute; National Institutes of Health. Effects of recruitment maneuvers in patients with acute lung injury and acute respiratory distress syndrome ventilated with high positive end-expiratory pressure. Crit Care Med 2003;31:2592-7.

61. Morrow BM. Chapter 6: An investigation into the effects on lung dynamics of performing a lung recruitment manoeuvre after endotracheal suctioning in ventilated paediatric patients. *In:* An investigation into nonbronchoscopic bronchoalveolar lavage and endotracheal suctioning in critically ill infants and children. PhD Thesis, University of Cape Town, 2005; pp 6.1-6.49.

62. Heffner JE, Hess D. Tracheostomy management in the chronically ventilated patient. Clin Chest Med 2001;22:55-69.

63. Lloyd-Owen SJ, Donaldson GC, Ambrosino N, Escarabill J, Farre R, Faurox B, Robert D, Schoenhofer B, Simonds AK, Wedzicha JA. Patterns of home mechanical ventilation use in Europe: Results from the Eurovent survey. Eur Respir J 2005;25:1025-31.

64. Jardine E, O'Toole M, Paton JY et al. Current status of long term ventilation of children in the United Kingdom: Questionnaire survey. BMJ 1999;318:295-9.

Ultrasound-guided Percutaneous Dilatational Tracheostomy

Alan Šustić

Percutaneous dilational tracheostomy (PDT) is an increasingly popular bedside technique in intubated, critically ill ICU patients that has generally low risks and appears to be cost effective. PDT is an invasive, semi-blind technique that relies on surface markings for correct identification of the anatomy. Portable Ultrasound (US) and endoscopy are the aids that can improve the safety of this procedure. The US offers a number of attractive advantages compared with competitive imaging techniques or endoscopy for imaging critically ill patients. It is widely available, portable, repeatable, relatively inexpensive, pain-free and safe. Although the earliest reports dealing with US applications in clinical medicine include the description of soft-tissue imaging of the pretracheal structures and anterior tracheal wall,[1] the first detailed reports of using US to assist in (percutaneous) tracheostomy date from the end of last decade.[2,3] Clinicians initially described US-guided central venous and arterial catheterization, followed by US-guided regional anesthesia techniques.

ULTRASOUND ANATOMY OF THE UPPER AIRWAY

For ultrasound analysis of the upper airway the most suitable probes are those with a small physical footprint (typically vascular or small parts probes) with higher frequency (> 7.5 MHz) and high resolution. The upper airway consists of the oral (nasal) cavity, pharynx, larynx and trachea, all of which are nearly completely air-filled. Due to the very high acoustic impendence of air, US cannot directly depict the inside of air-filled organs. Fortunately, due to their superficial position, the frontal and lateral walls of nearly all upper airway segments are visible by US examination either partially or completely. Using US we can image the floor of oral cavity and its lateral wall. The lateral wall, so called bucea appears as thin, hyperechogenic lines with a thin muscular layer underneath. We usually image only the second and third part of tongue as well as the base, while the anterior (frontal) third is examined only if the tongue is hard-pressed to the floor of the mouth.[4] For US imaging of the tongue and oral floor we use diagonal and vertical sections from top of mandible to hyoid bone. The US images show tongue as muscular organ with a typical hypo (-iso) echoic ultrasonographic structure; on both sides of the base, the valleculae are clearly visualized (palatopharyngeal fold), indicating the transition from oral cavity to the hypopharynx. In a lateral section, the hypoechoic tonsils are visualized, which especially in childhood, appear as lymphatic tissue with visible lateral walls of hypopharynx below. The lateral walls of nasal cavity are presented only in rare occasions when maxillary sinuses are filled with liquid.[5] The larynx is a musculocartilaginous structure situated below hyoid bone, formed by nine cartilages, the most important being the thyroid and cricoid. Both are very clearly visible by US as hyperechoic structures reciprocally connected by isoechoic membranous ligaments with visible air below. The ring shaped trachea, located inferior to the cricoid cartilage, is easily visible by US in longitudinal (Fig. 19.1) or transversal (Fig. 19.2) section together with the pretracheal tissue.[6] The trachea and paratracheal soft tissues of the neck can be examined with US probes of the highest frequency due to their superficial position. The anterior tracheal wall, thyroid and cricoid cartilages, tracheal rings and pretracheal tissue may all be well visualized, and allows the clinician to select the optimal intercartilagineous space for tracheostomy tube placement.

The relationship of the thyroid gland and the vascular structures of the neck to the trachea can also be readily seen on diagnostic US. Using US, Bertram and colleagues[7] found that in 15% of cases, the common carotid artery was less than 10.5 mm from the fourth tracheal ring and warned that the neck extension necessary for PDT can bring these vessels closer to the upper tracheal rings. Hatfield and Bodenham[8] found that two of their 30 patients had carotid arteries in the immediate paratracheal position, making them vulnerable to the consequences of non-midline placement of the needle and dilators, whilst another two had prominent brachiocephalic arteries. Half of the patients had anterior jugular veins and eight were near the midline at considerable risk, necessitating appropriate 'safety measures'. In their study, portable ultrasound provided a simple method of screening of vulnerable blood vessels in the neck and for locating the midline before percutaneous tracheostomy. As a patient-safety related practice, patients with unfavorable anatomy for PDT

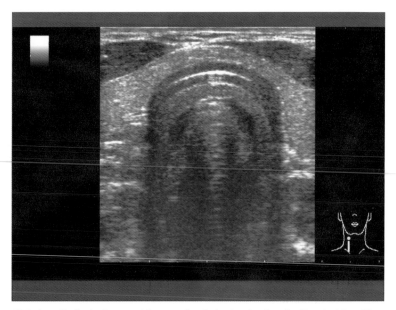

Fig. 19.1: Longitudinal ultrasound image of anterior tracheal wall with cricoid cartilage and tracheal rings (II – second; III- third)

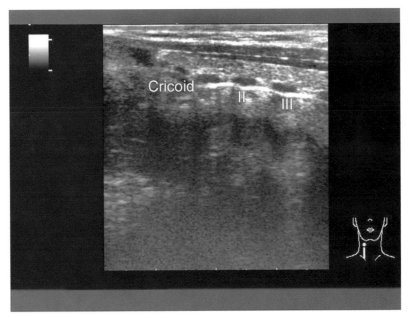

Fig. 19.2: Transversal ultrasonographic section of the anterior neck and trachea

demonstrated by US can be referred for open tracheostomy.

The Technique of Ultrasound-guided Percutaneous Tracheostomy

The PDT is an established and safe means of gaining tracheal access in intensive care.[9-11] However, the "blind" technique has significant potential complications and relative and absolute contraindications. To reduce these complications bronchoscopic or US guided PDT is suggested. Although bronchoscopic guidance is more often used and provides the best visualization, it has some disadvantages versus US. First, bronchoscopy is not without complications of its own, including compromised ventilation and significant hypercarbia with elevation of intracranial pressure, which could be distressing in patients with acute severe head or spinal cord injury.[12-15] Second, it was found that during bronchoscopy minute volume is significantly

reduced and that bronchoscopy "per se" could be responsible for pulmonary barotrauma and pneumothorax, a serious determent in the treatment of critically ill patients.[12,16] Third, bronchoscopy does not give any information about the presence of blood vessels or other structures outside the trachea and does not exclude possibility of serious bleeding incidents.[17] And finally, with bronchoscopy is not always possible to select optimal space between tracheal rings for tracheostomy. Despite the endoscopic guidance throughout the procedures, Dollner et al found, only 32% of the puncture sites were in the desired place.[18] On the other hand, using US guidance, cranial misplacement of tracheal tube, even in difficult cases, can be entirely avoided.[19] For this reasons, we and others have recently recommended ultrasound-guided puncture of trachea, a method that can be successfully used in all difficult cases.[2,3,20,21]

To perform US-guided PDT, though the author routinely uses a guide-wire dilatational forceps technique (Portex Ltd, UK), any of the PDT kits may be used. US-guided PDT is performed at the patient's bedside in the ICU using continuous physiologic monitoring. Ultrasonography can be especially useful to assess tracheal midline, pretracheal soft tissues, type and size of blood vessels in the area of interest, the strap muscles and the sternocleidomastoids, and more laterally the carotid arteries and jugular veins prior to PDT. After administering analgesia, sedation, and muscle relaxants, the patient is placed on 100% oxygen (FiO_2 of 1.0) and is prepared for PDT in a standard manner with or, if is it not possible, without neck hyperextension. With a linear transducer that has been prepared in a sterile sheath (we use short vascular probe, 5 - 10 MHz), the trachea is imaged in vertical medial section and the continuous Doppler signal over the trachea on the level of the second ring (or pulsed Doppler signal with sample volume in trachea) is activated. To decrease the chance of non-visualization of veins, the patient may be temporarily placed in Trendenlenburg position (head-down) to increase venous filling pressures in the region of interest. Care is taken during the screening to maintain only minimal pressure with the ultrasound probe to avoid obscuration of vascular structures by probe pressure. When round, well demarcated structures are identified anterior to the trachea that are suspicious of being vascular in nature, several maneuvres are applied to investigate whether the structures seen are veins or arteries. First, compression is applied with the probe to look for luminal narrowing in response to varying degrees of compression. Second, a Doppler curser is placed over the structure of interest and Doppler flow is displayed graphically and audibly to screen for evidence of pulsatile or low frequency flow signals typical of arteries or veins. Third, a square region of interest is placed around the structure and color Doppler analysis is performed.

The patient is in tracheostomy position, the endotracheal tube is thereafter withdrawn until the cuff is just below the vocal cords. When the tip of the tube reached the second tracheal ring, the intensity of the Doppler signal increases greatly due to an increased signal from unencumbered, turbulent air, confirming the correct position of endotracheal tube.[12] The site of puncture is usually selected between 2nd and 3rd tracheal ring, following a clear ultrasonic verification of anatomy of the thyroid and cricoid cartilage and tracheal rings. If the thyroid isthmus is situated alongside planed puncture canal we do not try to avoid it, since isthmus penetration is relatively frequent in PTD, but without serious consequences.[22] Then the ultrasound transducer is pulled cranially until the lower edge of transducer is placed above the tracheal ring, below which the tracheal puncture will be performed. After infiltration of anesthesia (local anesthetic with adrenaline), a transverse 1–2 cm long incision into the skin and subcutaneous tissue is made parallel and as close to the lower edge of transducer as possible. Then, the distance from probe to the echo of anterior tracheal wall is measured and marked on the cannula to be used for puncture. In order to control the depth of the puncture, we have designed special "stopper", consisting of a metal device, which avoids inadvertent injury to the posterior tracheal wall.[23] This stopper is positioned 5 mm distally from the indicated location on the cannula, and the puncture is performed through the incision up to the depth permitted by the stopper. Proper insertion into the trachea is verified by aspiration of air into a syringe attached to the cannula. After placing the guide-wire through the cannula into the trachea the cannula itself is removed. A 14-G dilator is then passed over the guide-wire to start the stoma formation. Then the guide-wire dilatational forceps is advanced along the guide-wire and tracheal stoma dilatation is performed as shown in Grigg's technique (see Chapter 7). Once adequate size of tracheal stoma is formed the forceps is removed and the tracheostomy tube is advanced along the guide-wire through the stoma into the trachea.

The correct position of tracheostomy tube is also confirmed at the end of procedure by means of US. [24-26] If the tracheostomy tube is in the correct position (i.e. in the trachea), bilateral equal motion of the diaphragm toward the abdomen is seen by sub-xiphoid or subcostal ultrasound imaging, representing equal bilateral expansion of the lungs. Conversely, if the tube is out of trachea, this will result in an immobile state of diaphragm during the positive pressure ventilation. Further an intercostal US view can identify "lung sliding" signs, a kind of "to and fro" movements of pleura synchronized with ventilation. If this sign is visualized on the left or on both sides of the chest it correlates with bilateral lung ventilation and with correct tracheostomy tube position.

There is growing body of literature demonstrating the value of ultrasonography in the care of critically ill patients, including central venous line placement and airway management.[27] The increasing availability of small, portable, competitively priced, ultrasound devices with high-resolution have lead to its increased use in intensive care setting. Ultrasonography is very useful and exact supporting method for PDT which could be an alternative to endoscopy in avoiding potentially serious complications of "blind" PDT.

REFERENCES

1. Katz AD. Midline dermoid tumors of the neck. Arch Surg 1974;109:822-3.
2. Šustić A, •upan •. Ultrasound guided tracheal puncture for non-surgical tracheostomy. Intensive Care Med 1998;24:92 [letter].
3. Muhammad JK, Patton DW, Evans RM, Major E. Percutaneous dilatational tracheostomy under ultrasound guidance. Br J Oral Maxillofac Surg 1999;37:309-11.
4. Neuhold A, Fuhwald F, Balogh B, Wicke L. Sonography of the tongue and floor of the mouth. Part I: Anatomy. Eur J Radiol 1986;6:103-7.
5. Lichtenstein D, Biderman P, Meziere G, Gapner A. The sinusogram, a real time ultrasound sign of maxillary sinusitis. Intensive Care Med 1998;24:1057-61.
6. Šustić A. Role of ultrasound in the airway management of critically ill patients. Crit Care Med 2007;35 (suppl):S173-7.
7. Bertram S, Emshoff R, Norer B. Ultrasonpgraphic anatomy of the anterior neck. J Oral maxillofac Surg 1995;53:1420-4.
8. Hatfield A, Bodenham A. Portable ultrasonic scanning of the anterior neck before percutaneous dilatational tracheostomy. Anaesthesia 1999;54:660-3.
9. Holdgaard HO, Pedersen J, Jensen RH, et al. Percutaneous dilatational tracheostomy versus conventional surgical tracheostomy: A clinical, randomized study. Acta Anaesthesiol Scand 1998;42:545-50.
10. Heikkinen M, Aarnio P, Hannukainen J. Percutaneous dilatational tracheostomy or conventional surgical tracheostomy? Crit Care Med 2000;28:1399-402.
11. Freeman BD, Isabella K, Cobb JP, et al. A prospective, randomized study comparing percutaneous with surgical tracheostomy in critically ill patients. Crit Care Med 2001;29:926-30.
12. Reilly PM, Sing RF, Giberson FA, et al. Hypercarbia during tracheostomy: A comparison of percutaneous endoscopic, percutaneous Doppler, and standard surgical tracheostomy. Intensive Care Med 1997;23:859-64.
13. Bardell T, Drower JW. Recent developments in percutaneous tracheostomy: Improving techniques and expanding roles. Curr Opin Crit Care 2005;11:326-32.
14. Kerwin AJ, Croce MA, Timmons SD, et al. Effects of fiberoptic bronchoscopy on intracranial pressure in patients with brain injury: A prospective clinical study. J Trauma 2000;48:878-82.
15. Hickey R, Albin M, Bunegin L, Galineau J. Autoregulation of spinal cord blood flow. Is the corda microcosm of the brain? Stroke 1986;17:1183-9.
16. Rudolf J, Neveling M, Gawenda M, Grond M. Pneumothorax following percutaneous dilatational tracheostomy. Clin Intensive Care 1998;9:136-8.
17. McCormick B, Manara AR. Mortality from percutaneous dilatational tracheostomy. A report of three cases. Anaesthesia 2005;60:490-5.
18. Dollner R, Verch M, Schweiger p, et al. Laryngo-tracheoscopic findings in long-term follow-up after Griggs tracheostomy Chest 2002;122:206-12.
19. Šustić A, Kovaè D, •galjardiæ Z, et al. Ultrasound-guided percutaneous dilatational tracheostomy: A safe method to avoid cranial misplacement of the tracheostomy tube. Intensive Care Med 2000;26:1379-81.

20. Šustić A, Krstuloviæ B, Eškinja N, et al. Percutaneous dilatational tracheostomy vs surgical tracheostomy in patients with anterior cervical spine fixation: Preliminary report. Spine 2002;27:1942-5.

21. Šustić A, •upan •, Antonèiæ I. Ultrasound-guided percutaneous dilatational tracheostomy with laryngeal mask airway control in a morbidly obese patient. J Clin Anesthesia 2004;16:121-3.

22. Šustić A, •upan •, Krstuloviæ B. Ultrasonography and percutaneous dilatational tracheostomy [letter]. Acta Anaesthesiol Scand 1999;43:1086-7.

23. Šustić A, Kovaè D, Krstuloviæ B. Ultrasound-guided puncture of trachea with «stopper»: A new supporting device for percutaneous tracheostomy. Eur J Anaesthesiol 2004;21 (suppl. 32):177-8.

24. Hsieh KS, Lee CL, Lin CC, et al. Secondary confirmation of endotracheal tube position by ultrasound image. Crit Care Med 2004;32(suppl.): S374-7.

25. Lichtenstein D, Menu Y. A bedside ultrasound sign ruling out pneumothorax in the critically ill; lung sliding. Chest 1995;108;1345-8.

26. Chun R, Kirkpatrick AW, Sirois M, et al. Where's the tube? Evaluation of hand-held ultrasound in confirming endotracheal tube placement. Prehospital Disaster Med 2004;19:366-9.

27. Guillory RK, Gunter OL. Ultrasound in the surgical intensive care unit. Curr Opin Crit Care 2008;415-22.

Chapter 20

Tracheostomy Tubes, Decannulation and Speech

Sushil P Ambesh

There are two primary types of tracheostomy tubes: cuffed and uncuffed. Cuffed tracheostomy tubes are used predominately for patients who require long-term ventilatory support or protection of their airways against aspiration because of swallowing (bulbar) problems. The uncuffed tracheostomy tubes are desirable because they allow exhaled air to pass through the upper airway enabling the individual to speak. The tubes can be disposable, usually made of PVC plastic or silicone, or nondisposable, made of metal, such as silver or stainless steel. Both cuffed and uncuffed tracheostomy tubes are available with or without inner cannulas. Inner cannulas are available in reusable and disposable types, and are removed for periodic cleaning, or if need be, for immediate clearing of secretions blocking the airway while keeping the artificial airway in place.

SELECTION OF TRACHEOSTOMY TUBE

There are no research data available documenting optimal choices in tracheostomy tube selection. However, while selecting the tracheostomy tube one should take in consideration the size, shape and composition of the tracheostomy tube according to patient's neck anatomy and problems. The size of the tracheostomy tube (TT) is described in terms of internal diameter (ID) of the tube in millimetre (mm) at its narrowest point. Tracheostomy tube must fit the airway and the functional needs of the patient. The diameter of the tracheostomy tube should be selected to avoid damage to the tracheal wall, to minimize work of breathing, and promote translaryngeal airflow when the cuff is deflated. If the tube is too small it will lead to increase in airway resistance and in turn increase in work of breathing during spontaneous respiration.[1] Small tube is quite vulnerable for frequent blockage with thick sticky secretions; in addition makes the suctioning of secretions more difficult. Further, small diameter tube will require increased cuff pressure to create a satisfactory seal against air-leak and that may increase the risk of ischemic injuries to the tracheal mucosa. If the tube is too large it may be difficult to insert through percutaneous approach and lead to problems with insufficient leakage past the tracheal cuff when cuff is deflated during weaning for spontaneous respiration (Fig. 20.1).

The curvature and length of the tube vary with size, designs and manufacturers (brand). The radius of curvature of the shaft of the tracheostomy tube should leave the axis of the distal portion of the tube in a collinear position with the axis of the

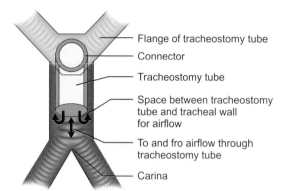

Flange of tracheostomy tube

Connector

Tracheostomy tube

Space between tracheostomy tube and tracheal wall for airflow

To and fro airflow through tracheostomy tube

Carina

Fig. 20.1: Tracheostomy tube in relation to tracheal lumen

patient's trachea. Appropriate positioning of the tracheostomy tube within the trachea can be determined either radiographically or by direct visualization with flexible bronchoscopy. Trachea is essentially a straight structure; anterior two third is rigid cartilaginous while posterior one-third is soft membranous that lies just anterior to esophagus. If the tube has pronounced curvature then the tip may get compressed against the anterior tracheal wall causing partial obstruction while middle portion of the shaft exerting more pressure on posterior tracheal wall. Longer tracheostomy tube is required in obese patients and patients with tracheomalacia or other anatomical abnormality. In majority of patients the tracheostomy tube should extend at least two centimeters beyond the stoma and no closer than 1-2 cm to the carina. Shorter is better than longer for most patients. The patients who are short statured and have short neck may be comfortable with smaller length of tube as normal length tube may stimulate the carina repeatedly and cause cough.

All tracheostomy tubes should be fitted with a 15-mm universal adapter to allow connectivity with Ambu bag or tubing connector for ventilation. Metal tubes are uncuffed and do not have this connector; therefore can not be used for controlled ventilation.

Most of the manufacturers supply tracheostomy tube with an obturator or introducer to aid insertion through tracheal stoma while avoiding the injuries

to mucosa with the tip of the tube. Double cannula tubes are supplied with an inner tube, which can be removed leaving the outer tube *in situ* and replaced after cleaning. Thus, incidence of life-threatening tracheal tube obstruction may be avoided. The main drawback of double tube is increase in airway resistance and work of breathing due to reduction in inner diameter of the tube. These double cannula tubes may be fenestrated or unfenestrated with a connector that fits with 15 mm ventilator tubing. The fenestrated tube has single or multiple openings in the posterior part of the outer tube. In a cuffed tube the fenestration lies just above the cuff. Deflation of the cuff of a fenestrated tube, while patient is breathing spontaneously, allows air to pass caudally through the tracheostomy lumen and fenestration, as well as around the tracheostomy tube, and up through the larynx. The fenestration allows maximum airflow through the larynx during speech and assessment for decannulation or down-sizing of the tube. If the patient is on controlled ventilation then unfenestrated inner tube should be placed in order to prevent air leak above the cuff.

TYPES OF TRACHEOSTOMY TUBE

PVC Tube

Shiley tracheostomy tubes (Tyco Healthcare, USA) are double cannula tracheostomy tubes with reusable inner cannula and twist-lock connectors. These tubes have a radiopaque, biocompatible outer cannula constructed of polyvinyl chloride (PVC). A Swivel neck plate allows conformity to individual neck anatomies. Shiley tracheostomy tubes are available in four sizes; 4, 6, 8, and 10. The cuffed tracheostomy tubes have thin walled, high volume low pressure cuff. The fenestrated tubes have a white 15 mm cap and a reusable fenestrated inner cannula with green 15 mm twist-lock connector (Fig. 20.2). The red decannulation plug can be used to occlude the proximal end of the outer cannula, forcing the patient to breath through the

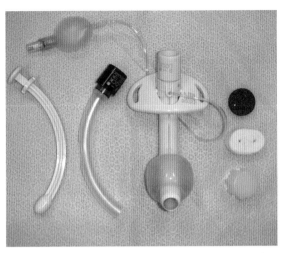

Fig. 20.2: Shiley fenestrated tracheostomy tube, unfenestrated inner tube *in situ* (white connector), fenestrated inner tube (dark green connector), tube tie, obturator, and cap (red and white)

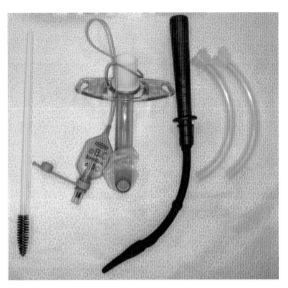

Fig. 20.3: Blue Line Ultra Tracheostomy Tube (Non USA), introducer (purple), two inner cannulas and a cleaning brush (supplied with single dilation percutaneous tracheostomy kit; Portex UK)

fenestrations and the upper airway tract during the weaning process. The manufacturer of the Shiley tube recommends its use not to exceed 29 days.[2]

The soft seal cuffed tracheostomy tube (Portex, UK) is supplied with two inner cannulas and an introducer. The introducer has a tunnel to accommodate the guide wire. This tube may be used for controlled ventilation for longer duration.

Portex Blue Line Extra Length Tubes (Fig. 20.3) are also available that have two independently inflated cuffs on the lower end of the extended length tube that allow flexibility in sealing the tube in alternate locations, or increasing the seal by inflating both cuffs at the same time.

Silicone Tube

The silicone tubes have more flexibility than the PVC tubes and may provide better fit, especially in some children whose individual anatomy presents problems in finding a good fit. The Bivona Aire-cut adjustable neck flange hyperflex[TM] tracheostomy tube (Fig. 20.5) is a radiopaque wire reinforced silicone tube with an inflatable silicone cuff and an inflation balloon with one way valve. It also

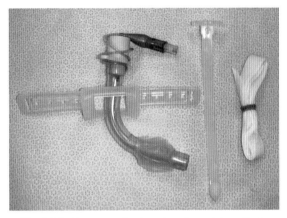

Fig. 20.4: Vygone cufferd tracheostomy tube with its introducer and adjustable flange

possesses 15 mm swivel and a sliding lockable neck flange. There is locking mechanism on the flange to maintain the correct tube length. The tube has measurement marks through out its length to determine the exact length of insertion for a particular patient. This tube provides temporary airway access for a tracheostomized patient and for the use in hospital care only, not for home use.[3]

The cuff pressure must be monitored periodically because diffusion of air through silicon cuff will cause slow deflation over time. The tube must be replaced with a fixed neck flange tracheostomy tube when the optimal length is determined. As the tube is wire reinforced, it should not be used during magnetic resonance imaging and laser surgery around the face and neck. These tubes are available only in single lumen without inner cannula; there is a greater risk of tube obstruction by secretions and therefore pure humidification of inspired gases should always be ensured.

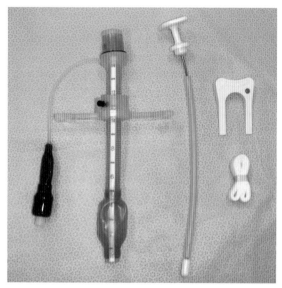

Fig. 20.5: Bivona tracheostomy tube with its introducer (Portex, Inc. Indiana, USA)

Mini-tracheostomy tube is an uncuffed tube (4 mm inner diameter) that is inserted through the cricothyroid membrane puncture using Seldinger guide wire technique (Fig. 20.6). This tube is especially useful to establish rapid access to the trachea, to facilitate suctioning of tracheal secretions and weaning. The tube is not for patients who require mechanical ventilation or who have impaired respiratory reflexes. The tube may be used for insufflations of oxygen to enrich the air in spontaneously breathing patients.

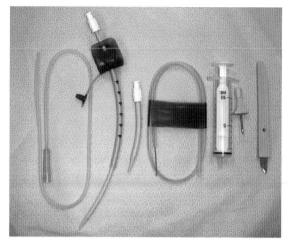

Fig. 20.6: Mini-tracheostomy kit showing 4 mm tube with accessories (Portex, UK)

CHANGE OF TRACHEOSTOMY TUBE

There are no definite guidelines describing the time interval for change of tracheostomy tube. Often, it is done on as and when required basis. At our institute we do it every fortnightly to prevent mucous build-up and to maintain cleanliness, unless contraindicated. However, change of tracheostomy tube within a week of tracheostomy formation is not warranted unless it is required due to compelling reasons. Following the tracheostomy, formation of tracheocutaneous tract takes about 10 days and after this period changing the tracheostomy tube generally poses no problem. Changing the tube within first week of tracheostomy may be associated with failure to recannulate the tract due to rapidly shrinking stoma after tube removal. Passing a bougie or airway exchange catheter before removal of existing tube may act as a guide for railroading the new tube. During the first change, all necessary equipments for endotracheal intubation must be at bedside and it should only be performed by the physician who is good in airway management. Change the tube before a feeding or at least 2 hours after the feed. All patients should be administered oxygen at least for five minutes, through the existing tube as well as face mask (if tube is partially blocked). In the event of failure to recannulate the tracheostoma, endotracheal intubation should be performed without further wasting the time.

DECANNULATION CRITERIA AND STRATEGIES

Keeping the tracheostomy tube for a long may expose patients to an increased risk of late complications, including tracheal stenosis, bleeding, fistulas, infections, tracheomalacia, tracheocele, aspiration and psychological or personality problems.[4-9] Removal of a tracheostomy tube is a fundamental step as well as the requirement in a rehabilitating patient recovering from critical illness.[10] Most patients are suitable for weaning as their condition improves. Limited uncontrolled pilot studies[11,12] and expert guidelines[13] have proposed that decannulation be considered in patients once respiratory mechanics are adequate, mechanical ventilation is no longer needed, upper airway obstruction is resolved, airway secretions are controlled and swallowing ability has returned. However, there are no definite guidelines and clinicians differ to reach common consensus criteria for tracheostomy decannulation. Recently, Stelfox et al conducted an international survey to find out determinants for tracheostomy decannulation, to establish a definition of decannulation failure and acceptable rate of tracheostomy decannulation failure.[14] According to their survey, clinicians rated level of consciousness, ability to tolerate tracheostomy tube capping, cough effectiveness and control of secretions as the four most important determinants in the decision to decannulate a tracheostomized patient. Patient comorbidities, etiologies of respiratory failure, swallowing function, respiratory rate and oxygen were judged to be of moderate importance. Age of the patient was rated as irrelevant. Previous studies and guidelines have suggested that maximal expiratory pressure, peak cough flows, arterial blood gases,

and upper airway endoscopy may be useful in the decannulation decision-making process; however, these factors require special equipments and expertise.[11-13]

While there is no consensus and defined protocol, many strategies for tracheostomy weaning have been suggested; however, a systemic multi-disciplinary approach, based on individual patient's haemodynamics and ongoing progress, has shown to improve likelihood of success.[15] Various methods of weaning that are practiced include increasing periods of cuff deflation, the use of fenestrated tubes and speaking valves, downsizing and intermittent capping of the tracheostomy tube prior to its removal. We, at our institute, practice intermittent deflation of cuff and downsizing of tracheostomy tube. If the patient tolerates the cuff deflation then a uncuffed tube or small size cuffed (deflated) tube is inserted. It is important that initial tracheostomy tube change must be performed by an anesthesiologist/ intensivist who is expert in airway management. Subsequent tube change may be done by respiratory care practitioner with a specific physician's order. For patients who effectively mobilize secretions without the need for suctioning for 24 hours, and successful completion of tracheostomy tube plugging for 24-48 hours, the tube may be removed. Documentation of decannulation must be made. Following tracheal decannulation the stoma is cleaned and covered with sterile dressings. Approximation of edges of tracheal stoma skin by suturing is generally not required. Physiological closure of tracheal stoma occurs within 24 to 48 hours; however, anatomical closure may take one week or more. Rarely, a small tracheocutaneous fistula may persist for a long time and that may require surgical closure.

Decannulation Failure

Tracheostomy decannulation is not without risk and there is currently no acceptable definition.

Extubation failure is defined as the need to reinstate mechanical ventilation within 24 to 72 hours of planned extubation.[16-18] Tracheostomy decannulation failure is defined as need to reopen the tracheostomy or perform endotracheal intubation because of an acute episode or progressive worsening of arterial blood gases not corrected by the application of non-invasive mechanical ventilation. Most clinicians consider reinsertion of artificial airway within 48-96 hours following planned tracheostomy tube removal to constitute a decannulation failure with an acceptable failure rate of 2% to 5%.[14] If there are repeated decannulation failures, hemodynamics, respiratory parameters and nutritional status are reviewed; ENT or pulmonary medicine doctors are consulted.

SPEECH

Deprivation of speech in a tracheostomized patient is a significant problem that hurts the patient psychologically, emotionally and socially. Studies have shown that speech in these patients acts as a psychological boost, allows communication and gives a feeling of general well beings. The relatives of the patient feel happy after hearing the voice of their closed one that encourages communication and social bonding. There are various methods to facilitate speech; however, all methods require deflation of tracheal cuff. While cuff is deflated, a part of expired air passes around the tube through the vocal cord apparatus. Occasionally, downsizing of tracheostomy tube is required to give enough space for airflow around the tube. A fenestrated tube allows maximal airflow. During this period the patient should be able to tolerate deflation without compromising the respiration and without the risk of aspiration. Alternatively, a one-way speaking valve may be attached with the tracheostomy tube to maximise the speech. The valve opens during inspiration to allow air to be entrained through the tube and closes during expiration to allow exhaled air to pass through the vocal cords to make phonation.[19] The valve then closes during expiration. The patients who are on ventilator, speaking valve may be employed to facilitate speech. Various types of speech valves are shown in Fig. 20.7.

Passy-Muir speaking valves can be used with air-filled cuffed tracheostomy tubes, but with great caution. The cuff must always be deflated when the Passy-Muir valve is in place in order to allow free exhalation through the upper airway. Use of Passy-Muir valve without deflating the cuff may cause lung injury and possible asphyxiation. Passy-Muir tracheostomy speaking valve with an uncuffed tracheostomy tube facilitates smooth speech both during inspiration and expiration, and also improves swallowing.

The Passy-Muir PMA 2000 Oxygen Adapter is small, lightweight, clear in color and easily snaps onto the PMV 2000 (Clear) and PMV 2001 (Purple) Valve. The PMA 2000 allows for easy delivery of supplemental low flow oxygen (<6 L/min) and humidity. Patients can improve their mobility and comfort by utilizing the PMA 2000 with oxygen tubing and a small portable oxygen tank, eliminating the need for bulky aerosol tubing. When using the PMA 2000, oxygen is delivered in front of the diaphragm of the PMV. This reduces complications associated with devices that provide continuous flow behind the diaphragm of a speaking valve which may include air trapping, drying of secretions and possible cilia damage.

The Passy-Muir PMV 2020 (Clear) (15 mm ID/23 mm OD) Tracheostomy swallowing and speaking valve is the only light weight one-way closed position "no leak" valve that attaches to the metal Jackson tracheostomy tubes (sizes 4 - 6 or equivalent) with use of the PMA 2020-S Adapter. The PMV 2020 (Clear) is intended for use by both short-term and long-term adult, pediatric and neonatal non-ventilator dependent tracheostomized patients.

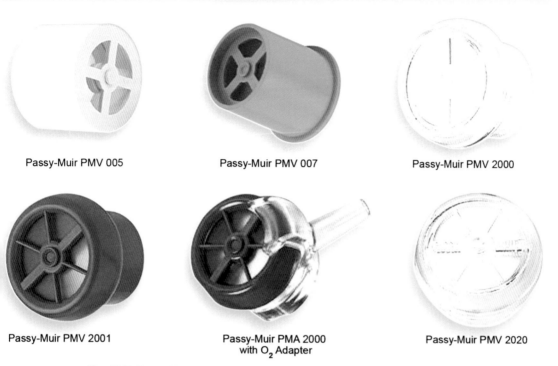

Passy-Muir PMV 005   Passy-Muir PMV 007   Passy-Muir PMV 2000

Passy-Muir PMV 2001   Passy-Muir PMA 2000   Passy-Muir PMV 2020
                              with O₂ Adapter

Fig. 20.7: Passy-Muir tracheostomy, ventilator, swallowing and speaking valves

Talking tracheostomy tubes are offered by uritan Bennett (Phonate™), Portex (Trach Talk Jue Line®), and Boston Medical (Montgomery® ENTRACH) to enable speech with an inflated uffed tube.

EFERENCES

1. Epstein SK. Anatomy and physiology of tracheostomy. Resp Care 2005;3:476-82.
2. Instruction insert for the Shiley tracheostomy tube. Tyco Healthcare Group LP, Nellcor Puritan Bonnet Division, Pleasanton, CA USA.
3. Instruction insert.
4. Epstein SK. Late complications of tracheostomy. Resp Care 2005;50:542-9.
5. Heffner JE, Miller KS, Sahn SA. Tracheostomy in the intensive care unit. Part 2: Complications. Chest 1986;90:430-6.
6. Dulguerov P, Gysin C, Pemeger TV, Chevrolet JC. Percutaneous or surgical tracheostomy: A meta-analysis. Crit Care Med 1999;27:1615-25.
7. Freeman BD, Isabella K, Lin N, Buchman TG. A meta-analysis of prospective trials comparing percutaneous and surgical tracheostomy in critically ill patients. Chest 2000;118:1412-8.
8. Norwood S, Vallina VL, Short K, Saigusa M, Fernandez LG, McLarty JW. Incidence of tracheal stenosis and other late complications after percutaneous tracheostomy. Ann Surg 2000;232:233-41.
9. Gilony D, Gilboa D, Blumstein T, Murad H, Talmi YP, Kronenberg J, Wolf M. Effects of tracheostomy on well-being and body image perceptions. Otolaryngol Head Neck Surg 2005;133:366-71.
10. Christopher KL. Tracheostomy decannulation. Resp Care 2005;50:538-41.
11. Ceriana P, Carlucci A, Navalesi P, Rampulla C, Delmastro M, Piaggi G, De Mattia E, Nava S. Weaning from tracheostomy in long-term mechanically ventilated patients: Feasibility of a decisional flowchart and clinical outcome. Intensive Care Med 2003;29:845-8.
12. Bach JR, Saporito LR. Criteria for extubation and tracheostomy tube removal for patients with ventilatory failure. A different approach to weaning. Chest 1996;110:1566-71.

13. Heffner JE. The technique of weaning from tracheostomy. Criteria for weaning: Practical measures to prevent failure. J Crit illn 1995;10:729-33.

14. Stelfox HT, Crimi C, Berra L, Noto A, Schmidt U, Bigatello LM, Hess D. Determinants of tracheostomy decannulation: An international survey. Crit Care 2008;12:R26.

15. Hunt K, McGowan S. Tracheostomy management in the neurosciences: A multidisciplinary approach. Br J Neurosci Nurs 2005;11:122-5.

16. Vallverdu I, Calaf N, Subirana M, Net A, Benito S, Mancebo J. Clinical characteristics, respiratory functional parameters, and outcome of a two-hour T-piece trial in patients weaning from mechanical ventilation. Am J Resp Crit Care Med 1998;158:1855-62.

17. Esteban A, Alia I, Tobin MJ, Gil A, Gordo F, Vallverdu I, Blanch L, Bonet A, et al. Effect of spontaneous breathing trial duration on outcome of attempts to discontinue mechanical ventilation. Spanish Lung Failure Collaborative Group. Am J Resp Crit Care Med 1999;159:512-8.

18. Epstein SK. Decision to extubate. Intensive Care Med 2002;28:535-46.

19. Hess DR. Facilitating speech in a patient with a tracheostomy. Resp Care 2005;4:519-25.

Index

Acute respiratory distress
          syndrome 19
Adam's apple 31
Adopt standard evaluation 127
Adrenaline solution 50
Advantages of
     percutaneous tracheostomy 20
     TLT method 73
Air embolism 28
Airway
     control 58
     fire 28
     management devices 90
     obstruction by foreign bodies 30
Alley's forceps 26
Ambesh T-trach 95
Amoxycillin 24
Anesthetic preparation and
          technique 92
Apnea 28
Apparatus and procedure 80
Arterial blood pressure 85
Artificial
     airways 18
     nose 137
Arytenoids cartilages 13
Atracurium 93
Balloon facilitated percutaneous
          tracheostomy 8, 80
Blind 151
Blood vessels ligature 32
Brantigan's and Grow's papers 29
Bronchial intubation 35
Bronchopneumonia refractory to
          treatment 19
Bronchopulmonary hygiene 53
Bulbar poliomyelitis 19
Burns 19
Button scar 20
Cadaveric position 15
Cannula
     adapter 66
     connector 66

exchange 60
insertion 61
placement 70
Cardiac arrest 28
Catheter
     mount 66
     over needle 31
Cervical
     spine clearance 113
     trachea 120
Changing of tracheostomy tube 27
Chest injury 19
Chronic
     bronchitis and emphysema 19
     pain 19
Ciaglia
     blue rhino tracheostomy (CBR)
          78
     dilators 95
     dolphin balloon 95
     kit 45
     technique 45, 53
Clauvulanic acid 24
Closed
     position 51
     versus open suctioning 141
Cochrane review 141
Complications of prolonged
          translaryngeal intubation 18
Cone-cannula 66
Consider respiratory function 126
Continuous
     electrocardiography 85
     endoscopy allows 58
     positive airway pressure 19
Contracture neck 107
Contraindications of percutaneous
          tracheostomy 107
Conventional tracheostomy 127
Count percentage of
          contraindications 128
Cricoid hook 25

Cricothyroideal membrane
          puncture 31
Crusts 28
Cuff inflation line 66
Cuffed
     oropharyngeal airway 91
     ventilation catheter 66
Curved needle 66
Decannulation
     criteria and strategies 159
     failure 159
Difficult tracheostomy 126
Difficulty of airway access 127
Dilation 59
Draping 24
Early postoperative 28
Emergency
     percutaneous tracheostomy 112
     transtracheal airway catheter 31
End tidal carbon dioxide 85, 96
Endotracheal
     suctioning 139
     tube 40, 68
Epiglottis cartilage 13
Esophageal
     obturator device 92
     perforation 35
Esophagus 15
Essential anatomical data of neck
          126
Evolution of
     cuffed tracheostomy tube 4
     percutaneous tracheostomy 6
Fantoni's translaryngeal
          tracheostomy 45, 112
Fiberoptic bronchoscope (FOB) 117
Fixation
     skin 117
     tape 66
Flail chest 19
Gastric aspiration 35
Glottic edema 19, 30
Grade C evidence 112

Granuloma formation 28
Griggs
  forceps 95
  technique 53
Guidewire
  and tracheostomy tube 10
  dilating forceps 8, 49
Guillain-barre syndrome 19
Head position 58
Heat and moisture exchanger 137, 138
Hematoma 107
Hemorrhage 101
High innominate artery 107
History of tracheostomy 1
Humidification 137
Humidifiers 138
Indications for
  suctioning 140
  tracheostomy 19
Infection 19
Inferior laryngeal nerve lesion 35
Injury to
  paratracheal structures 28
  trachea and larynx 28
Insertion of tracheostomy tube 26, 95
Inside percutaneous techniques 72
Instruments for tracheotomy 23
Intensive care unit (ICU) 18
Intra-operative
  complications 28
  hemorrhage 28, 35
Intrathoracic trachea 120
J wire 66
Kelly's forceps 8
Lancet 66
Largely obese patient 63
Laryngeal
  and subcricoid stenosis 19
  lesions 35
  ligaments 14
  mask airway 30, 91
  muscles 14
  tumors 23
Laryngotracheal stenosis 28
Larynx 12, 15
Lateral thyrohyoid ligaments 14
Learning and training 35

Lignocaine 24
Low pressure ventilation 31
Misplacement of tracheostomy
  tube 103
Mobilization of bronchial secretions 139
Monitoring 96
  of tube cuff pressure 143
Morbid obesity 111
Multiple
  dilatation technique 39
  organ system dysfunction 19
Muscle weakness 19
Myasthenia gravis 19
Needle
  insertion 58, 68
  puncture 31
Neurological disorders 19
Obturator 66
Operative technique 25
Operatory rooms 118
Outside/inside
  percutaneous 131
  tracheostomy 65
Oxygen saturation (SpO$_2$) 96
Part preparation 24
Patient positioning 24
Patil emergency cricothyrotomy
  catheter 31
PDT in special situations 111
Peak
  airway pressure 85, 96
  inspiratory pressure 67
Percutaneous
  cricothyrotomy 31, 34
  dilatational tracheostomy 23, 89, 111, 116, 149
  nephrostomy technique 56
  tracheostomy 46, 130
PercuTwist method 92
Perforation of posterior tracheal wall 103
Peripheral hemoglobin oxygen
  saturation 85
Pneumothorax 28, 103
Polyvinyl chloride (PVC) 156
Portable ultrasound (US) 149
Positive

end-expiratory pressure 40, 67, 108
  pressure ventilation 4
Possible variations of technique 72
Postoperative hemorrhage 35
Postoperatory tracheobronchial
  toilette 30
Post-tracheostomy chest X-ray 97
Preferred technique 67
Programmed
  decannulation 61
  replacement of cannula 76
Pull handle 66
PVC tube 156
Quadrilateral laminae 12
Randomized controlled trials (RCT) 117
Rate of ring fracture 128
Recruitment of collapsed alveoli 143
Relations of
  larynx 15
  trachea 16
Reliable index of local trauma 128
Repeat tracheostomy 112
Respiratory
  paralysis 19
  plethysmography 53
Rhino's horn 8
Rigid tracheoscope (RTS) 66
Rosary 65
Rotation difficulty 61
Safety
  measures 16, 150
  thread 70
Secondary hemorrhage 28
Securing tracheostomy tube 97
Seldinger
  guidewire 8, 34, 49, 80
  technique 6, 31, 44, 50
Selection of tracheostomy tube 155
Sellick's maneuver 13
Severe
  brain injury 19
  chronic obstructive pulmonary
    disease 19
  thrombocytopenia 115
Shiley tracheostomy tubes 156
Silicone tube 157

Single tapered dilator technique 42
Sinusitis 19
Skin incision 59, 116
Skull base fractures 30
Sodium chloride 141
Speech 160
Stage of dilation 70
Sterility 140
Subglottic stenosis 35
Suctioning technique 141
Superior
    and inferior thyroid arteries 15
    laryngeal
        artery 15
        nerve 15
Supraglottic airway devices 91
Surgical
    cricothyrotomy 31, 32
    emphysema 103
    preparation and techniques of PT
        93
    tracheostomy 116, 128, 130
Technical considerations of Ciaglia's
        techniques 43
Teflon catheter 45

Tetanus 19
Thyroid cartilage 12
Timing of tracheostomy 20
Trachea 15
Tracheal
    cannula 40
    dilatation 106
    necrosis 28, 102
    puncture needle 10
    stenosis 104
    wall incision 117
Tracheobronchial hemorrhage 30
Tracheocutaneous fistula 28
Tracheoesophageal fistula 28, 106
Tracheoinnominate artery fistula 105
Tracheomalacia 106
Tracheostomized patients 145
Tracheostomy 56
    cannula insertion 60
    scar 28
    tube 155, 158
Tracheotomy 56
Translaryngeal
    endotracheal tube 90
    intubation 18, 56

tracheostomy 65, 80
Transtracheal jet ventilation (TTJV)
        31
Trendenlenburg position 24
Trismus 30
Trousseau dilator 26
Tube
    blockage 28
    displacement 28
Tumor 107
    of larynx 19
Twill tape 27
Types of tracheostomy tube 156
Ultrasound anatomy of upper airway
        149
Uncuffed tube 34
Vacuum pressure 140
Vascular and nerve supply 15, 17
Vecuronium 93
Ventilation 72, 75
Water vaporizers 138
Work of breathing (WOB) 20
Wound infection 28
Yttrium-aluminium-garnet (Nd-YAG)
        105